Ophthalmic Echography

Cynthia J. Kendall, BMET

SLACK Incorporated, 6900 Grove Road, Thorofare, New Jersey 08086

Printed in the United States of America

Library of Congress Catalog Card Number: 87-42952

ISBN 1-55642-027-7

Published by: SLACK Incorporated
               6900 Grove Rd.
               Thorofare, NJ 08086-9447

Last digit is print number: 10   9   8   7   6   5   4   3   2

To my father
Raymond Kendall
who will always be
my guiding light

Contents

About the Author

Cynthia J. Kendall, BMET, has been active in the field of ophthalmic echography for over ten years. She received her degree in Biomedical Engineering Technology from Howard Community College in Columbia, Maryland. Beginning in 1980 as an electronic repair and installation technician for Xenotec, Ltd., in Frederick, Maryland, she rapidly learned about ophthalmology and ultrasound. This company specialized in the manufacture of A-scan and B-scan instrumentation.

After traveling throughout the country as a field service technician, she realized that many "service" problems were in fact "in-service" problems—that there was often a lack of understanding of how the equipment worked and what to do to produce a valid image. Her interest in eyes (her brother has diabetic retinopathy and she is myopic herself) led to extensive reading, studying, and questioning of physicians, technicians, and engineers regarding the subject of ophthalmology in general and ultrasound specifically.

This book is in part an integration of ideas developed while working with numerous echographers from around the world. For several years, she was the ultrasound product manager for Biophysic Medical. This French ophthalmic laser and ultrasound equipment manufacturer is now owned by Alcon Surgical. Since 1989, she has been an independent consultant. Her clients have included Alcon, 3M Vision Care, and Innovative Imaging, as well as a number of prominent medical institutions.

Throughout the years, she has taught many accredited courses for both JCAHPO (Joint Commission on Allied Health Personnel in Ophthalmology) and ASORN (American Society of Ophthalmic Registered Nurses). These courses have covered A-scans, IOL calculations, and B-scans. Since 1987, she has delivered the physics lecture at the annual ultrasound course for the Manhattan Eye, Ear and Throat Hospital in New York City.

The author has a sincere interest in encouraging ophthalmic medical personnel to better understand and appreciate the value of an echographic examination. After studying this book, the author trusts that readers will have many of their questions answered and will be launched into the fascinating world of echography.

Foreword

Cynthia Kendall has created an important addition to the field of ophthalmic ultrasonography—namely, a thorough overview of the field. Her down-to-earth review of each subject, while geared predominantly for the ophthalmic technician, will be of benefit to anyone interested in reviewing or extending their knowledge of ultrasonography. Cynthia writes the way she speaks, in a clear and straightforward fashion that is easy to understand. The information is derived from years of experience within the industry and an extensive period of clinically related exposure. She has participated in numerous academic teaching programs and has helped many technicians, physicians and related industrial individuals gain a perspective of this important field. I can recommend this book without reservation to all those interested in the field, recognizing that this work will surely be followed by additional comprehensive writings which will add to an incredible first effort.

Yale L. Fisher, MD
Chairman, Department of Ultrasonography
and Co-chairman, Vitreoretinal Service
Manhattan Eye, Ear & Throat Hospital;
Assistant Clinical Professor
Cornell University Medical Center

Acknowledgments

Now I know why so many authors say that they cannot thank everyone who helped make their book possible. It's true, but I'll try nonetheless. The person who first fired my interest and excitement about entering a new career was my professor, Bruce Reid. He made discovering the secrets of electricity an exciting adventure. I also wish to thank: Bill Lindgren, president of Xenotec, who always let me interrupt his thoughts with my unending questions; Marci Fishman, RDMS, who showed me my first clinical B-scan and standardized A-scan examinations at UCLA in 1980; Karl C. Ossoinig, MD, Sandra Byrne, and Ron Green, MD, who have kindly allowed me to be their shadow for years and years; John Shammas, MD, who always has a smile and a word of encouragement; Yale Fisher, MD, who finally got it through to me how to think three-dimensionally; the many physicians and technicians who not only asked me questions for which I had to find answers, but who answered mine and taught me many of the tidbits which I share with you in this book; Patrick Coonan, MD, for his kind offer of an examination room for a Saturday morning photo session; Michael Kelly, Director of Ophthalmic Photography at Pacific Presbyterian Medical Center for taking the examination technique photos; my family and friends who supported me during this monumental task, especially Wayne Bittinger, who did a terrific job of copy editing the manuscript; Jillian Giese, Larry Swenson, Helen Aragon, my Aunt Janey Bahle, and others who let me scan their eyes for the photos in this book; Kelly Chenik, the Macintosh wizard who created some of the illustrations; and last but not least, my publisher and editors at SLACK Incorporated, who have had enormous patience with me. I graciously thank you all.

Introduction

The purpose of this book is to provide an overall view of the field of ophthalmic echography, or ultrasound as it is also called. There are many different clinical applications of ophthalmic ultrasound technology. Some of these are: axial eye length A-scan biometry used in calculating intraocular lens (IOL) power; A-scan pachymetry for measuring corneal thickness; diagnostic B-scan for mapping intra- and extraocular structures such as the extent of a retinal detachment or the size and location of a tumor; and diagnostic A-scan for aiding in the differentiation of normal and abnormal structures.

An ophthalmic medical assistant may be in a position to use all or only one of these different modes of ultrasound. Although the basic principles may be learned from this book, the application of these principles in a clinical setting should be considered by the reader as the lab portion of this training. Practical suggestions and helpful hints will be offered throughout this volume, and additional suggestions that would complement future editions are welcomed.

HOW IT BEGAN

An unexpected series of events brought me to the position of writing a book to assist ophthalmic medical personnel in understanding and effectively using diagnostic ultrasound. Actually, my goal is more than just increasing understanding. It is also to share the excitement of this fascinating field and thereby inspire some of you to go on to become accomplished diagnosticians and teachers.

For me it all began in 1977 when I changed my career from clerk/typist to student of biomedical engineering technology (BMET). Immersed in the hectic schedule of classes and part-time jobs, there was absolutely no way for me to appreciate how many exciting avenues there were in the field of electronic medical instrumentation. Since that time, I have been privileged to work with many of the finest doctors, echographers, physicists, and engineers from around the world. They have been and still are my teachers and mentors. They have inspired me to learn and to never stop asking questions. I hope that through this book I can give back a part of what has been given to me.

There is a story I would like to share that was a highlight of my early career as an installation, training, and repair person of ophthalmic ultrasound instruments. It occurred in the spring of 1980 while driving across Kentucky on a very rainy Sunday afternoon. I stopped at a state park for a brief rest and met an older couple. We began talking and I explained that I worked with equipment used by eye surgeons. The woman said that her husband had been blind in one eye for over 35 years. He had been accidentally shot with a BB gun when he was a child. At that time, the doctor wanted to enucleate (remove) the eye. His family said no, and never again did he see an ophthalmologist. He even managed to get through military service without anyone noticing his visual deficiency; during physical exams he memorized the eye chart using his good eye.

I could not resist bringing out my penlight to look at his eye. The cornea was clear and through the torn pupil the lens appeared cloudy, as though he had a traumatic cataract caused by the BB that had damaged his iris and probably touched the lens. I was so curious that I asked a few more questions and even performed a little experiment. When he covered his good eye, he could tell the difference between a catsup bottle and a soft drink can that were next to each other on the table before him.

With only limited knowledge, this seemed to indicate to me that his retina had at least partial function. I have since come to realize that the phrase "I am blind" is a relative statement.

I told him, "I'm not a doctor, but I know that ultrasound is often used to examine someone who has your condition. When the sound waves from the ultrasound instrument are directed into the eye, they produce a picture in much the same way that a ship uses sonar to map the ocean floor. From this picture, the doctor can see how many structures in the eye are intact. With that information and some other tests, he can judge whether or not you might be able to have some sight restored through surgery."

When I arrived at my destination, the doctor for whom I was installing equipment agreed to see the gentleman who subsequently volunteered to be our subject during the in-service training. We performed axial eye length A-scans on both eyes and a diagnostic B-scan on the injured eye. Both tests showed that his eyes were normal except for the cataract and the tear in the iris.

The cataractous lens was removed, but an intraocular lens could not be implanted at that time due to the damaged iris. The cataract surgery was a complete success and with a contact lens, the patient now has a corrected vision of 20/20.

That experience, at the beginning of my career in medical instrumentation, made quite an impression on me. I realized just how far a little knowledge and interest can go. I am glad that I took the time to ask questions, listen to the answers, and share with this man some of the advances made in ophthalmology since his eye injury so many years before.

On that note, let us begin learning about what we can do to help patients receive the care and treatment they need in order to obtain the best possible vision and health.

The first thing to learn will be the most basic principles of echography. I know that you will be pleasantly surprised to learn that many of the things you already know about the properties of light will apply when learning about sound. The chapter devoted to principles will be followed by chapters discussing instrumentation and the various applications that may be encountered in the clinical setting. Case studies will be presented so that you may follow the thought processes used in determining the proper treatment for each patient.

CHAPTER 1

Ultrasound Principles

ULTRASOUND

The word ultrasound means ultrahigh frequency sound waves. These are above the audible hearing range—that is, they cannot be heard by the human ear. This concept encompasses a large range of applications. These include: prenatal scans, giving expectant mothers and their physicians details about the condition of the fetus; lithotripsy, using ultrasound to break up kidney stones; cardiovascular studies, providing vital information concerning the heart and arteries; and orthopedic use, relieving muscle strain.

In ophthalmology, the use of diagnostic ultrasound is not as well known to the general public as are these other specialties. Yet there is a vast amount of ophthalmic ultrasound knowledge to be shared. Our goals are to provide the best possible care for patients as well as to develop our own abilities and sense of accomplishment. This chapter will introduce you to basic principles critical to understanding how this examination method is used.

ECHOGRAPHY/ULTRASONOGRAPHY/SONOGRAPHY

Three different words are used interchangeably: echography, ultrasonography, and sonography. Since you will encounter all of these terms in various publications and educational courses, it is helpful to be familiar with their various word forms and pronunciations.

1. Echography, Ultrasonography, Sonography:
   The making of an image using sound waves
2. Echographer, Ultrasonographer, Sonographer:
   One who performs patient examinations using ultrasound
3. Echogram, Ultrasonogram, Sonogram:
   The image produced by ultrasound

The following is a listing of these words with the apostrophe (') mark indicating the syllable that should receive the most accent:

E-chog'-ra-phy
E-chog'-ra-pher
Ech'-o-gram
Ul-tra-son-og'-ra-phy
Ul-tra-son-og'-ra-pher
Ul-tra-son'-o-gram
Son-og'-ra-phy
Son-og'-ra-pher
Son'-o-gram

The words echography and ultrasonography are used in ophthalmology; sonography is most often used in body scanning, which is generally part of a radiology department.

WHAT YOU ALREADY KNOW

The first thing to realize is that you already know more about ultrasound than you might think. You know how light behaves and this knowledge may be applied to ultrasound. If you can imagine what a ray of light would do, then you can imagine what the invisible ultrasound beam does when it enters an eye.

Think of the ultrasound probe as sending out a sound beam just like a flashlight sends out a beam of light. In our application the sound beam is very small and can be precisely directed toward ocular structures. Like light waves, ultrasound waves can bounce off of surfaces, reflecting back some of the energy. They can also be focused, absorbed, or refracted by a lens or other structure.

Knowledge of how light behaves may be directly applied to understanding how ultrasound behaves. It can be useful to imagine an ultrasound probe as a tiny "flashlight" that shines sound into the eye.

It is important to understand these basic principles so that the images to be interpreted will make sense. It is not enough to simply memorize certain patterns of A-scan and B-scan echoes, because there will always be exceptions. When the fundamentals are understood and applied, the operator will be able perform an examination with efficiency and precision. In doing so, the echographer will take his place as a vital member of the diagnostic team.

CLASSIFICATIONS

Before going further into the realm of the invisible sound beam, it is necessary to realize that the word ultrasound can mean different things to different people. Therefore, when talking about ultrasound, you must be certain that your listener understands which type is being discussed. Each type is used for entirely different applications and has significantly different effects on the tissues to which it is applied. The three classifications are:

1. Ultrasonic cleaners
2. Therapeutic ultrasound
3. Diagnostic ultrasound

Because of the major differences between these, it merits taking time now to be clear about how diagnostic ultrasound differs from the others. Three properties distinguish these classifications:

1. The generation or lack of generation of heat
2. The power of the sound energy (ultrasonic power) applied to the tissues, measured in watts per square centimeter (W/cm^2)
3. The frequency of the sound waves, measured in cycles per second or hertz (Hz)

Ultrasonic Cleaners

Ultrasonic cleaners are quite often found in or around an operating room. They are used to clean delicate instruments prior to sterilization. You may also have seen similar devices in a jewelry store. An ultrasonic cleaner is simply a bath of fluid (in a medical setting it would most likely be distilled water) which is made to vibrate so that molecules of water will knock off debris found on instruments. This is a very efficient method of cleaning. However, if you feel the water after a while, it will be warm. The first characteristic listed above, that of generation of heat, is an important one to note. This heat results from the second property, the power of the sound energy emitted. The third characteristic is frequency, which is relatively low here. Generally speaking, when used as a cleaner these high power sound waves are emitted at a rate of several thousand cycles per second, or kilohertz (kHz).

Therapeutic Ultrasound

Therapeutic ultrasound is used to treat a medical condition. It is commonly applied to ankles, knees, back, or any area of the body that has a muscle strain. When relieving muscle strain, the generation of heat from the relatively high ultrasonic power combined with the low frequency of the transducer allows the therapist to elevate the temperature of tissues in order to increase the blood supply and stimulate the lymph system to carry away excess fluid in the area of an injury.

A relatively new application is that of lithotripsy where a device aims a high power ultrasound beam at a kidney stone. The energy breaks the stone into small fragments to facilitate the patient passing them without pain.

There are two relatively new applications for therapeutic ultrasound technology in ophthalmology, treating glaucoma and melanoma. The temperature of tissues associated with glaucoma is elevated when the sound beam is directed toward them. A thermal effect, similar to laser, causes the trabecular meshwork to open up, allowing aqueous fluid to drain. This procedure is performed as a last resort treatment for patients who are not responding to more conventional therapies. Studies are also being made to determine the effectiveness of using this high power ultrasound to treat malignant melanoma.

Diagnostic Ultrasound

Now we arrive at the area that is of greatest interest to those wanting to learn more about A-scans and B-scans. Diagnostic ultrasound is significantly different in all three properties from the previous two categories.

Diagnostic ultrasound as used in ophthalmology is in a class by itself. It is quite different from the kind used in ultrasonic cleaners, or the therapeutic type used in physical therapy for an injured muscle.

1. It does not generate heat in the ocular tissues.
2. It does not use high power sound energy.
3. Its frequency is much higher, in the range of millions of cycles per second, called megahertz (MHz).

These properties lead us to a very important conclusion: Diagnostic ultrasound is a safe and effective method of generating ocular images for all types of patients. This is especially true because there is no radiation or magnetism associated with ultrasound.

MORE TERMINOLOGY

The terms ultrasound and echography have already been defined in this chapter. There are some additional terms, some of which have meanings in applications different from A- and B-scans, while others may apply only to this field of study. The following definitions will accent the usage of terms as they apply to ophthalmic echography. Once they have been defined, principles that affect scanning will be outlined.

Frequency

As has been discussed earlier in this chapter, frequency is a numeric value for the number of cycles per second. The unit of measure is the hertz, abbreviated Hz. You will see another letter in front of the Hz when we talk about ultrasound. For example, the figure 10 MHz, a common frequency for ophthalmic ultrasound probes, indicates that the sound beam is being generated at a rate of 10 million cycles per second or 10 megahertz. The higher the frequency of an ultrasound probe, the less deeply its sound can penetrate into the tissues. Therefore, high frequencies are used in the eye whereas lower frequencies such as 2.5 MHz and 5 MHz are used in body scanning.

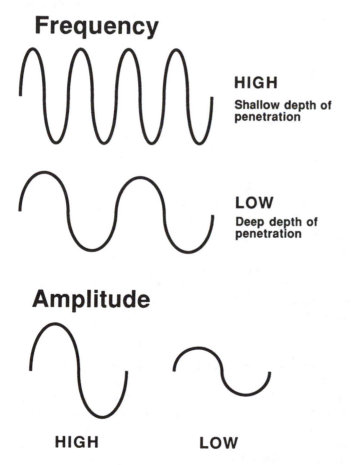

Figure 1.1 Frequency and amplitude are both important properties of ultrasound.

Resolution

Resolution is a word commonly used to define the quality of an image in terms of its spatial elements. Even though this is quite a subjective area, the difference between a high resolution image and a low resolution image is fairly obvious. To put it very simply, an image is designated as high resolution if it can show the separation between two or more very closely spaced objects. The resolution of an imaging device is specified as a unit of distance, in our case millimeters. This value is related to the wavelength and frequency of the sound energy as well as the design of the electronic components within the imaging instrument itself.

It is important to realize that the higher the frequency, the shorter the wavelength and therefore the better the resolution. This relationship between frequency and resolution is fundamental because it is the reason why we can obtain clear images of tiny ocular structures. It is this basic physical principle that determines the resolution capabilities of any ultrasound imaging device.

A high-resolution image simply means one in which small objects that lie closely together are visualized. In ophthalmic echography, some instruments produce high-resolution images capable of resolving an optic nerve cup of only 0.7 mm.

Velocity

Velocity is a word related to speed. There are two reasons why we need to understand at what speed the sound is traveling through certain ocular tissues:

1. To obtain accurate measurements
2. To interpret artifacts (unwanted echoes)

In order to make accurate measurements of ocular structures, we must know through what structures and at what speed the sound is traveling. Each structure has its own characteristic density which will change the speed of sound in that structure. This is important because there is enough of a difference in the densities of the various ocular structures to affect the accuracy of the measurements. A measurement is calculated by using the following simple formula:

Distance = Time (seconds) × Velocity (meters/second)

Ultrasound systems do not directly measure the distance between structures, they merely measure the time it takes for each echo to be returned from a structure to the probe. Once the time interval has been recorded, the value is multiplied by the appropriate velocity for the type of structure being measured. The resulting distance value is usually automatically displayed on the instrument's screen.

The word propagation is also used when discussing the speed of sound through a given tissue. The following is a list of velocities of propagation used in our application:

1532 m/s	Aqueous and vitreous humor
1548 or 1550 m/s	Average for axial eye length measurements
1550 m/s	Soft tissue
1620 m/s	Cornea
1641 m/s	Crystalline lens

There has been much discussion over the years about the specific velocity of sound through the lens. Since the lens structure can be significantly changed by the development of a cataract, it is logical to suspect a change in the velocity as well. And this is indeed the case. However, it is nearly impossible to visually observe a cataractous lens and then make a judgment as to the amount the velocity would change. Therefore, the value of 1641 m/s is considered to be the most accurate. There are some instruments that may use a velocity of 1620 m/s. The slight difference of 20 meters per second when measuring a structure that is about 3–5 millimeters in thickness has a negligible effect. At the 1988 meeting of SIDUO (the International Society for Diagnostic Ultrasound in Ophthalmology), held in Argentina, a new paper was presented showing that recent research supports earlier findings of a lens velocity of 1641 m/s.

Transducer

The transducer is the most amazing part of an ultrasound unit, truly the heart of the system. Originally, transducers were made from a type of quartz crystal. In our application, it is a small ceramic plate that sends out sound waves when energized by an electrical pulse. The part of the ultrasound system that sends the electrical pulse to the ceramic is called the transmitter. Following a short electrical excitation pulse, the very same ceramic receives or "hears" the reflected sound waves and converts them into electrical signals to be displayed on a screen.

The piezoelectric ceramic plate transducer that sends and receives sound waves is truly an incredible device. This ceramic device is the foundation of every ultrasound system in the world.

The piezoelectric (pronounced "pee-yay'-zo-e-lec'-tric") effect is the name for this incredible feat of nature. In its generic form, the word transducer refers to any device that converts energy from one form to another. A piezoelectric transducer converts electricity to sound waves and sound waves to electricity, thereby making it possible for diagnostic ultrasound to be performed.

When it is built into a device, the transducer is called a

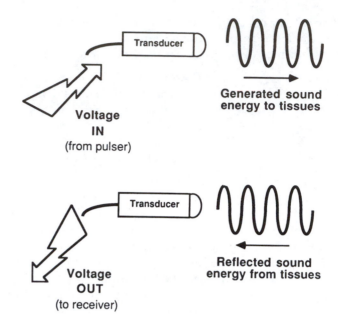

Figure 1.2 Ultrasound transducers are ceramic plates that transform electricity into sound waves and sound waves into electricity.

probe. Sometimes the actual ceramic comes into direct contact with the eye, as in the case of a solid-tipped A-scan probe. Other times it is recessed inside a fluid-filled probe. A stationary transducer is used for A-scans and a larger, motorized, fluid-filled probe is used for B-scans.

Signal Processing

What happens to the echoes the transducer hears? The part of the ultrasound system that gathers the returned echoes is called the receiver. The receiver sends the signals to a signal processor to prepare them for being displayed.

Figure 1.3 shows a series of echo patterns. The first one approximates the tiny echo as it is received by the probe. Next it is amplified. Then the lower half of the wave form is cut off. This is called detection. A line is drawn connecting the tops of each wave and this is called an envelope. The echo is amplified once more and finally displayed on the screen.

The purpose of describing this sequence of events is to demonstrate that a great deal of work is done to the tiny received echo long before it ever appears on the screen. This signal processing should be considered as the key determining factor in how the echoes appear on the screen. It is what makes each manufacturer's piece of equipment produce an image that is different from the others.

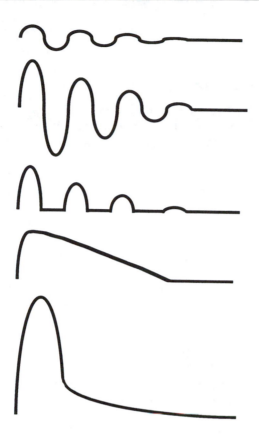

Figure 1.3 The echo seen on the display barely resembles the initial echo received by the transducer. Signal processing makes the echoes easier to interpret. The top drawing simulates the actual echo as received by the transducer. The bottom echo simulates the echo as it is seen on a display. In between are the stages of processing.

Imagine making an audio recording of someone whispering. Now imagine how it might sound if you played that recording loudly enough for a person on the second balcony of a concert hall to hear. There would certainly be a lot of distortion, as when the volume of a stereo is turned up too loud. This is the sort of problem that engineers have to solve when designing a system that can amplify and yet let us see the reflected echoes from the eye without excessive distortion and noise.

Gain

Gain is an electronic amplification of a sound wave signal that is received by the transducer. This amplification factor is called the decibel, abbreviated dB. It is also quite common to use the word sensitivity when referring to this concept. Really, this is quite easy to remember. When the gain is turned up, the A-scan echoes get taller and the B-scan echoes get brighter. Conversely, when the gain is turned down, the echoes get shorter and dimmer. This is one of several factors that determine how the echoes will appear on the screen.

Sound Beam Characteristics

There are two characteristics of a sound beam to be considered here. First, there is the shape of the beam. Sound beams are said to be focused or unfocused. The focused beam is generally used in axial eye length A-scan probes and the B-scan probes. The point of maximum focus is usually designed to be near the retina of an average length eye. The unfocused parallel beam is used in standardized diagnostic A-scan probes and often in generic diagnostic A-scan probes. To focus a sound beam, a lens is placed on the tip of the ceramic transducer, much as a lens might be placed in front of a flashlight beam.

A second characteristic of a sound beam is that it may be defined in terms of its width. An effectively wide beam is used to first produce an echo during a diagnostic exam, while an effectively narrow beam is used to make accurate measurements. The reason for using the word effective is to show that the beam does not actually get wide or narrow when the gain is turned up or down. What we are doing to the image when varying the gain is to selectively choose how much of the echo we wish to have displayed.

A radio station can send out a very powerful signal from its transmitter. The amount we choose to listen to is determined by our adjustment of the volume control. In addition, when the volume is turned up too loud, the resulting distortion makes it difficult to understand the words of a song. A volume too low will also result in an inability to

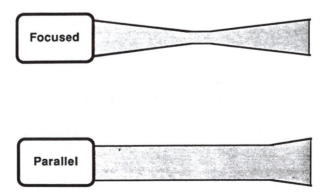

Figure 1.4 The shape of a sound beam can be altered with a lens to focus or defocus it; left alone it tends to be parallel. Focused beam probes are used in axial length and B-scans, while unfocused parallel beam probes are used for diagnostic A-scans.

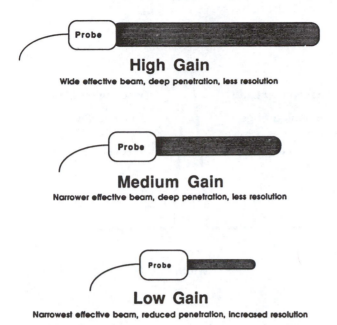

High Gain
Wide effective beam, deep penetration, less resolution

Medium Gain
Narrower effective beam, deep penetration, less resolution

Low Gain
Narrowest effective beam, reduced penetration, increased resolution

Figure 1.5 Although the actual amount of sound energy going into the eye does not change, the effective increase and decrease is made by adjusting the gain. Although high gain can decrease resolution, (the ability to see two small things close to each other) it does increase sensitivity (the ability to see echoes from weak sources such as vitreous membranes). Low gain has more resolution and less sensitivity.

understand. Similarly, a gain level on an ultrasound unit that is too high or too low may allow you to see echoes, but not necessarily allow the echoes to be properly interpreted.

Ophthalmic ultrasound uses a fixed energy system, whereas other forms of body scanning may utilize equipment that allows the operator to adjust the amount of sound energy that is being directed into the tissue. It is interesting to note that the Food and Drug Administration (FDA), which limits the power levels for medical imaging applications, allows a significantly smaller amount of sound energy to be used in ophthalmic scanners than is permitted in fetal scanners.

If the energy of the sound beam going into the eye is fixed, why change the amount of echo that is displayed? Adjusting the gain will allow us to vary the resolution, or sharpness, of the image. Remember that resolution is the concept of how close together two things may appear and still allow you to discriminate both objects.

In the clinical application, when examining a retina that may be totally detached, turning down the gain will effectively narrow the beam, thereby increasing the resolution and guiding you to the determination of whether the macula is still attached or not. For a traction detachment patient, a high gain will allow better visualization of the membranes which pull on the retina, but a reduced gain will again

Sound beams may be manipulated like light. B-scan and axial length probes focus the sound energy to increase its usefulness and effectiveness.

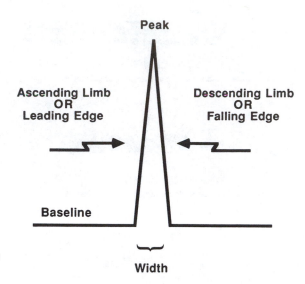

Figure 1.6 Each A-scan echo can be described by referring to its various parts.

increase the resolution and help locate the exact point of traction so that the retinal surgeon may know exactly where to treat the condition.

There is no single setting of gain that is correct for all conditions. The sensitivity will be varied throughout an examination depending upon the specifics of the case and the particular tissues of the eye to be imaged.

Anatomy of an Echo

The line at the bottom of the echoes on the display screen is called the base line. The A-scan echoes rise up from this point in varying heights. As they begin to rise, the left edge of the echo is called the ascending limb, or leading edge. When the echo reaches its highest point, it is at its peak. On the way back down to the base line, the terms applied to the echo are descending limb, or trailing or falling edge. Echoes may also be described in terms of their width. This is the distance between the points of attachment to the base line of the ascending and descending limbs.

Artifacts

Artifacts are usually considered to be unwanted echoes that do not represent ocular structures. They can truly be confusing at times because although they are real echoes, they do not represent actual tissues. In chapters 4 and 6, additional examples of artifact images will be given. Mention is

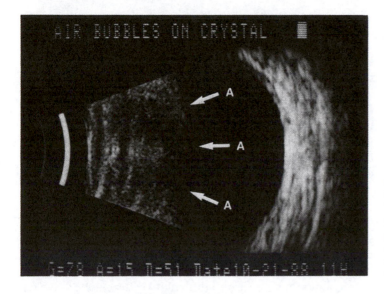

Figure 1.7 In probes filled by the user, micro bubbles on the face of the crystal can cause noise artifacts in the anterior portion of the image and an overall reduction of sound energy. This indicates the need to clean and refill the probe.

made here, however, because one of the most common instigators of artifacts for the echographer is the presence of an air bubble in the pathway of the sound beam. Since ultrasound does not travel through air, the bubble can be a problem.

Unwanted air bubbles may be in the probe itself, in the coupling medium, or even in the eye as in the case of a penetrating injury or pneumatic retinopexy. Pneumatic retinopexy is a treatment for retinal detachment that involves injecting air into the eye in order to help reattach the retina.

Air bubbles are the nemesis of ultrasound. During all echographic examinations, one must be constantly on the lookout for them.

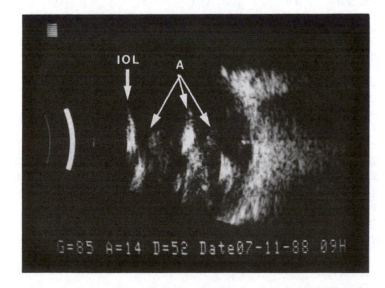

Figure 1.8 The presence of an intraocular lens (IOL) can cause confusing echoes in the vitreous space on both A- and B-scans. The extra echoes are caused by reverberations of sound that is reflected by the IOL.

Artifacts are unwanted echoes caused by scattering, reflection, and reverberation. Sometimes they can be useful clues to the nature of the object that could have created them.

Air in the eye will act as a reflector of the sound waves; consequently, there will be only a very bright echo on the screen followed by a shadow, or lack of all echoes. This bright echo is produced by the interface between the ocular tissues and the air bubble. No clinical ultrasound information beyond that bubble will be visible on the screen. Depending upon the size of the bubble, however, the patient's head may be positioned in such a way as to allow the bubble to be moved away from one area for scanning. The patient can then be asked to move his/her head into another orientation for the examination of additional areas. The thing to remember, of course, is that the bubble will tend to rise, making the superior retina the most difficult to examine.

Artifacts created by air bubbles inside the A-scan or B-scan probe indicate that the probe needs to be cleaned and refilled.

Air is such a strong reflector that in the case of a penetrating injury it is sometimes difficult to differentiate between a small air bubble and a foreign body in the eye. Foreign bodies are often made of glass or metal, which are also strong reflectors of sound—in fact, so strong as to prevent ultrasound imaging of the tissues posterior to the object. This image would show a very bright echo from the foreign body, and a shadow behind it. A shadow may cause either a partial or total loss of echo signals posterior (to the right on the screen) to the foreign body.

Another type of artifact is reverberation. Sometimes sound will bounce back and forth inside an object in the eye, resulting in a series of echoes behind the one from the initial encounter with the object. Usually these are produced by foreign substances such as glass shards, pellets from a BB gun, steel fragments, or the plastic of an intraocular lens (IOL).

In the case of a BB, there is a characteristic comet tail appearance to the chain of echoes that follows the initial echo from the surface of the steel. This is the result of the spherical shape of the pellet.

On several occasions, I have been sent photos produced by B-scan equipment that supposedly had a problem. As it turned out, the real problem was the difficulty of trying to scan through an IOL. The acoustic impedance (the difference between the aqueous and the artificial lens material) is so great that significant reverberation echoes are produced. This gives the appearance of a serious vitreous pathology or perhaps something wrong with the probe.

From these examples, it is easy to see that knowledge of artifacts and how they might be caused can lead to more effective scanning techniques and more reliable diagnoses.

FACTORS INFLUENCING HEIGHT AND BRIGHTNESS

Besides manually adjusting the gain, there are three factors which influence the height of an A-scan echo or the brightness of a B-scan echo. These are:

1. The angle of the sound beam when it encounters a structure
2. The relative difference between two tissues
3. The size and shape of the interface between tissues

Sound Beam Angle

The first factor in influencing the height and brightness of an echo is the angle at which the sound beam encounters the ocular structure to be imaged. This angle is called the angle of incidence.

Imagine standing in front of a mirror with a flashlight pointed directly at the mirror. There would be a 90 degree angle of incidence resulting in reflected light so bright that it would be uncomfortable to your eyes. If the angle that the light strikes the mirror is less than 90 degrees, then a large amount of the light will be reflected in another direc-

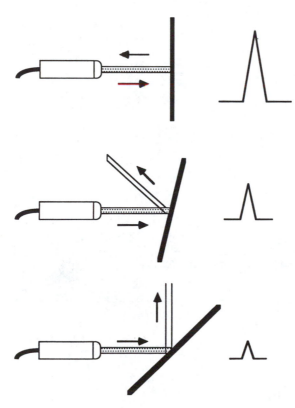

Figure 1.9 When the sound beam is directed perpendicularly to a structure, the maximum amount of sound will be reflected back to the probe. When only five degrees off axis, the echo will be zero in the case of a physical reflector. In the case of a biological reflector, there may be a small reflection even when slightly off axis due to a scattering effect.

The angle at which a sound
beam encounters an ocular
structure is called the angle of
incidence. This is an important
property to understand since
the probe that sends sound
waves into the eye must also
be in the correct position to
receive echoes.

tion. The more the flashlight is tilted away from the perpendicular position, the less the light will be visible. At 90 degrees, the flashlight itself will "see" all of the reflected light. Once the angle is no longer 90 degrees, then the light bounces off in another direction, not back toward the source.

Sound waves behave in exactly the same way. Since the probe is both sender and receiver of the signal, the key to optimal detection is to position the probe so that its transmitted wave is perpendicular to the structure to be imaged. In summary, the maximum amount of reflected sound will be obtained when the sound beam from the probe is directed at a 90 degree angle to the tissue. The farther away from this ideal angle, the lower in amplitude the resultant echo will be.

Interfaces Between Tissues

The second factor influencing the height and brightness of an echo is the relative difference between the various tissues the sound beam encounters. Each time the sound beam passes from one kind of tissue into another, a certain amount of energy will be reflected back toward the probe. If there

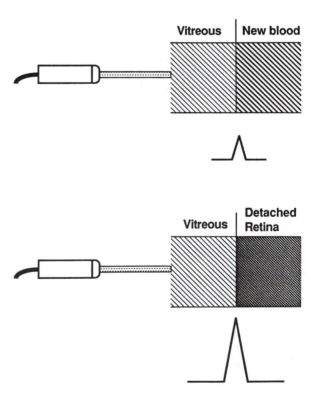

Figure 1.10 When
perpendicular to an interface,
the quantity of reflected sound
will depend on the amount of
dissimilarity between the
tissues. Similar tissues reflect
only a little, while dissimilar
ones reflect more.

is a substantial difference between the tissues, there will be a substantial echo. Conversely, if there is only a small difference between the tissues, then only a small echo will be displayed. This is assuming that the sound beam is perpendicular to the interface of dissimilar tissues.

The term for this property is acoustic impedance. Acoustic, of course, refers to sound, and impedance has to do with how easily or how well something moves. Therefore, it can be said that the difference in acoustic impedance between vitreous and new blood is very slight resulting in a small echo, whereas the difference between a detached retina and the vitreous is great producing a large echo. Remember that these are strong or weak echoes due to the significance of the tissue interface. In both cases, the sound beam is still perpendicular to the interface.

When two similar tissues lie next to each other, they may not produce much of an echo, even if the sound beam is directed toward them perpendicularly. However, if the difference between them is great, then the resultant echo will be strong.

Texture and Size of Interfaces

The third factor influencing the height and brightness of an echo deals with the texture and size of the interface. A smooth interface like a retina will allow some of the energy

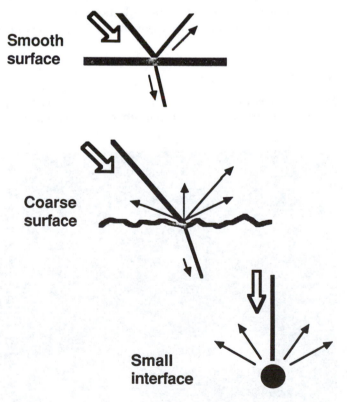

Smooth surface

Coarse surface

Small interface

Figure 1.11 The smoothness and size of a structure can also influence the amount of sound energy being reflected by an interface.

A-scan

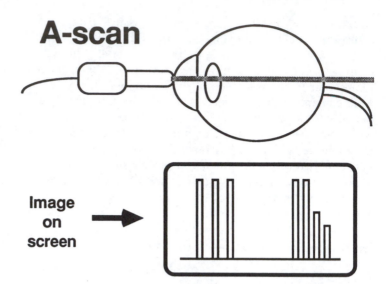

Image on screen →

Figure 1.12 The stationary transducer in an A-scan produces a one-dimensional display.

It is easier to obtain a strong echo from a smooth tissue like the retina, than from a coarse structure like the ciliary body.

to pass through while reflecting only part of it. A coarse surface, like a ciliary body or a membrane with folds, tends to scatter the beam, sometimes without providing any single strong reflection. Some of the energy will also be transmitted through a coarse surface. In addition, a small interface produces a scattering of the reflections, whereas a larger interface can reflect a greater portion of the sound energy.

A-SCAN

What then is an A-scan? It is a one-dimensional display from which clinical judgments are made based on the ampli-

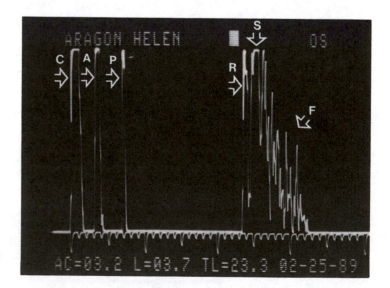

Figure 1.13 The characteristic echoes in an axial eye length A-scan are cornea (C), anterior lens (A), posterior lens (P), retina (R), sclera (S), and orbital fat (F).

tude and spacing of echoes. Hence the A in A-scan is for amplitude. The transducer is "stationary"—that is to say that although the examiner may move the probe, the probe itself has no moving parts.

If an echo is tall on an A-scan, it will produce a bright spot on a B-scan. Conversely, short echoes on A-scan appear as dim echoes on B-scan.

B-SCAN

The B-scan on the other hand is a two-dimensional display from which clinical judgments are made based on the various levels of brightness of echoes. Here is where B-scan gets its name—B for brightness. The design of a B-scan probe is really quite an amazing feat of engineering. The crystal inside the B-scan probe moves back and forth constantly in order to send an array of sound beams into the eye. Having the little crystal oscillate so quickly and both send and receive the echoes requires very precise timing.

The A in A-scan stands for amplitude, because we judge the echoes according to their height. The B in B-scan stands for brightness, since we judge the echoes according to their level of brightness.

The relationship between A- and B-scan echoes is that structures which produce a tall echo on an A-scan will produce a bright echo on a B-scan.

When I first heard that a B-scan was made up of hundreds of A-scans lined up in sequence one above the other, it didn't make any sense at all. I could see that some instruments had the ability to display an A-scan at the bottom of the image of a B-scan. This simultaneous A-scan is called a vector, or a cross-vector line. On the B-scan image, there is a black or white line going from left to right through the scan indicating the place from which the A-scan on the bottom of the screen came.

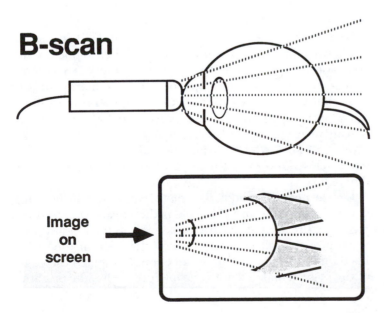

B-scan

Image on screen

Figure 1.14 The moving ceramic inside the B-scan probe sends out an array of individual sound beams. The reflections from each beam is organized and displayed as a two-dimensional image.

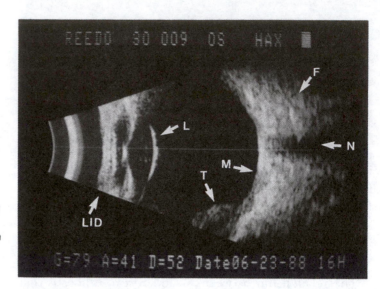

Figure 1.15 This B-scan directed through the horizontal axis of the eye shows the eyelid (LID), posterior lens (L), a tumor (T), the macula (M), optic nerve (N), and orbital fat (F).

After having it explained to me, I could see that when the vector line was positioned on the B-scan through a bright, white part of the picture, the spike, or echo, on the A-scan was pretty tall. If the line went through a black area of the image there was no echo on the A-scan at all. Pale or dim parts of the B-scan showed up as small echoes on the A-scan. Now the relationship between tall echoes on A-scan being similar to bright echoes on B-scan started to make sense. But really, how could a stack of A-scan images be turned into a B-scan picture?

One way to understand this concept is to picture a thick book. Imagine that someone has written their name on the edges of the pages while the book was closed. If you look at any one page, there would be little ink marks on the edge, but without the other pages, you could never figure out what was written. This is a perfect analogy with how a B-scan image is created using many A-scans. Each page represents an A-scan and the edges of the pages when the book is closed represent the display screen of the ultrasound device.

Lay the imaginary book flat and turn it so that the binding is away from you and then open the cover. On the first page, picture an A-scan with its base line at the binding and the top of the tallest echo touching the edge of the page. Each time the A-scan echo is tall enough to reach the edge of the page, it makes a dot. The taller the echo, the brighter the dot. When there are no echoes on the A-scan, there are no echoes on the B-scan either, and that area is black.

REQUIREMENTS FOR SUCCESS

There are two aspects of performing a successful ultrasound examination that cannot be underestimated. These are patience and patients.

Patience

Patience is required at all times during the process of evaluating an eye with echography. Careful thought and consideration must be given to the instrument settings, the direction of the sound beam, and the interpretation of the spikes and dots on a screen. The popular aphorism applies here: Patience is a virtue. Of course, patience with patients is more than essential.

Patients

The patient with a known pathology can be one of the greatest teachers of all. They will open the doors to understanding. And even if there are no patients available who require scans, it is expected that technicians and physicians practice on themselves. When you create a scan of your own eye (through a closed lid) the iris, posterior lens capsule and optic nerve should all be centered on the display. When scanning yourself you will appreciate the need for tiny, gentle probe movements. You may then truly say to the patient, "I have had this test myself and I understand what you will be experiencing."

CONCLUDING REMARKS

A periodic review of this chapter will allow these concepts to become unconsciously understood. As time goes on, you will notice that you often do not consciously think about what to do next—the hand/probe movement will be automatically made, adjusting the orientation of the sound beam, resulting in the desired image quality on the screen. Imagining what the sound beam is doing inside the eye will help provide positive results. In addition, there are three important principles especially worth remembering:

1. The high frequency ultrasound that is the basis for ophthalmic echography does not travel through air.

(There is no way around this one. There simply must be no air in the pathway of the sound.)
2. The maximum reflected echoes will be produced when the sound beam is perpendicular to the structure.
3. The larger the difference between the materials at an interface, the greater the reflected sound energy.

CHAPTER 2

Clinical Applications

A POWERFUL DIAGNOSTIC TOOL

There are several different situations in the course of the treatment and care of an ophthalmic patient that may call for a diagnostic ultrasound examination. Having such a powerful and safe diagnostic tool at one's fingertips can greatly enhance any clinic or practice by providing specific and detailed information regarding the anatomical structures of the eye. This information enables the physician to provide the best possible treatment and care for a large variety of ocular disorders.

In an office where only one type of ophthalmic ultrasound is available, it is still very important to understand the role of the other modalities as well. At some point during the course of treatment, a patient may require additional scans and it will be valuable to know where the patient may be referred and for which additional scans. It is the purpose of this chapter to provide an overview of the many different applications currently available, thus enabling the reader to assist in the proper management of the patient.

In later chapters, each application will be discussed in greater detail with specific examination techniques demonstrated. The types of ophthalmic echography described here are:

1. Axial eye length A-scan
2. Corneal thickness pachymetry A-scan
3. Contact diagnostic B-scan
4. Standardized echography

A-SCAN AXIAL EYE LENGTH MEASUREMENT

The most frequently used type of ultrasound in ophthalmology today is the axial eye length A-scan used to measure the eye prior to cataract surgery. This is just one of many types of A-scan used in ophthalmology. A synonym for this type of A-scan is biometry. Many people simply say that

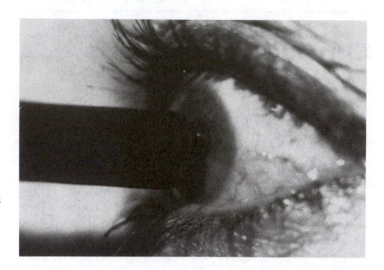

Figure 2.1 An A-scan probe is gently placed against an anesthetized cornea, directing the sound beam along the visual axis.

A-scan used for measuring the axial length of an eye prior to IOL implantation is the most common type of echographic examination performed. This is a type of biometric scan.

the patient needs to have a biometry, or that an ultrasound needs to be performed. To be more specific, the phrase "the patient requires an axial eye length measurement" would be preferred. Actually, the word biometry does not specifically have to do with ophthalmology. It is merely a term used when discussing biological data and statistics. Other common usages of the word are seen in "biometric" A-scan, and in referring to the ultrasound unit itself as a "biometer."

This type of measurement of an eye's axial length pro-

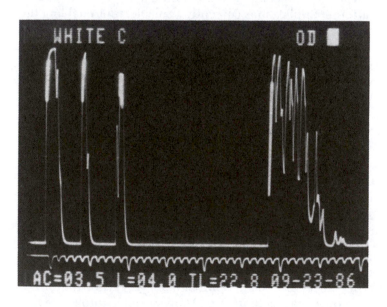

Figure 2.2 A classic axial eye length A-scan displays echoes from cornea, lens surfaces, retina, sclera, and orbital fat. Under the scan are displayed values of anterior chamber depth (AC), lens thickness (L), and total length (TL).

vides one of the three important values needed to calculate the appropriate power of an intraocular lens (IOL) implant. Refer to the chapter on IOL calculations for a more in-depth discussion of the part axial length plays in this calculation.

There are several other reasons why an axial length measurement might be performed even when cataract surgery with IOL implantation may not be planned. These are:

1. Preoperative scanning of both eyes for evaluation of similarities or differences
2. Postoperative verification of eye length
3. Postoperative determination of anterior chamber depth
4. Verification of aphakic spectacle refraction
5. Documentation of eye growth patterns

Preoperative Scanning of Both Eyes

Even if surgery is only required on one eye, it is customary to scan both eyes prior to performing cataract surgery with an IOL implantation procedure. This additional information is very useful for both the examiner and the surgeon. If the eyes are of considerably different lengths (more than 0.3 mm), the patient's chart must be reviewed for information such as the oldest known refraction that would support such a finding. It is fairly unusual for a person to have eyes that are significantly different from each other with respect to their refractive errors. Therefore, if the measurements are not similar between eyes, you should expect to see that the patient has a difference in the refractive errors corresponding to this length difference.

Since both eyes in a patient are usually very similar, scan both and compare the measurements. If they are not within 0.3 mm of each other, repeat the scan. Read the patient's chart to look for old spectacle refractions that justify why the eyes are of different lengths.

A difference may also be found in the keratometer readings, measurements of the corneal curvature. When in doubt, measure both eyes again to be certain that they are in fact dissimilar, then notify the surgeon of your findings. This difference may affect the IOL power chosen, since it is important to consider the refraction of both eyes when making the decision of which power to choose. Refer to chapter 8 for more information regarding the effects of axial length, corneal curvature, and natural lens power.

Postoperative Verification of Eye Length

There are two reasons for scanning an eye after an IOL is already in place. Unfortunately, there are times when the postoperative refraction differs from the surgeon's expectations. The first step in looking for the reasons is to examine the original axial length A-scan. It may not have been correct. This is easy enough to confirm by simply repeating the scan. Chapter 4 will outline special considerations to be mindful of when performing these scans.

After surgery, a postoperative axial length measurement may provide a clue to understanding the cause of unexpected results.

The second situation that may require the scanning of a pseudophakic eye (an eye with an IOL rather than a natural lens) occurs when the patient's nonoperated eye has developed a cataract and is to undergo surgery. The operating surgeon may not have been the same one who performed the first surgery. In this case, measuring the eye with the IOL already in place provides an extra measure of security when it comes time to compare the lengths of both eyes. In addition, when an IOL is to be selected, it will be helpful to the surgeon to have every possible bit of data to take into consideration. For the examiner's confidence, the same rule applies in scanning both eyes for their similarity even when one of the eyes has an IOL.

Postoperative Anterior Chamber Depth

The postoperative measurement of anterior chamber depth (ACD) represents the distance between the anterior surface of the cornea and the anterior surface of the IOL. It is measured in millimeters and is a critical factor in making IOL calculations. However, there is no way of knowing the precise value prior to surgery. This means that the value entered into the IOL formula can only be an estimate based on the results of many other surgeons who entered into clinical trials for various IOL manufacturers.

The postoperative results from these clinical trial surgeons are tabulated, and it is these values that help the surgeons who come afterward. Such preliminary results provide an idea as to what might be expected with certain types of IOLs. However, after being surgically implanted, the IOL might end up in a slightly different position with respect to the cornea than was anticipated. This difference in position will translate into a difference in postoperative refraction.

A careful measurement of the pseudophakic eye will produce a postoperative value for the actual anterior chamber depth. This distance can be a very useful piece of information. In fact, the knowledge of the exact postoperative depth of an IOL can help the surgeon increase his or her accuracy of the predicted post-op refraction for future surgeries.

Verification of Aphakic Refraction

An unusual case involved a young patient who was aphakic (without a natural lens) and for whom a secondary IOL implantation was not planned. This child was mentally retarded and was unable to read the eye chart or to communicate. The physician performed a retinoscopy examination to determine what the aphakic spectacle power should be. For an interesting confirmation, the axial length A-scan and keratometry (K) readings were made and put into an IOL formula that also calculated aphakic spectacle refraction. This proved to be a useful method for double-checking the correct power for this child's glasses independent of her ability to tell the physician how well she could see.

Documentation of Eye Growth Patterns

There are two points of interest on the subject of documenting eye growth. One is that studies are being made which evaluate the eye length of children at various times to document normal growth patterns. The second point is that there have been studies of the axial eye lengths of children with glaucoma which show that their eyes are longer than normal for their age. This can be yet another piece of information that will help the physician to make the best possible diagnosis and develop the best possible treatment plan for children.

A-SCAN CORNEAL THICKNESS PACHYMETRY

Corneal thickness pachymetry (pronounced "pa-kim'-a-tree") is another type of biometric measurement performed with an A-scan. This knowledge has a variety of applications. Pre- and postoperatively, the thickness of the cornea may be one of the factors that can indicate the relative health of the cornea. For example, a thicker than normal measurement may show that the patient has edema (swelling caused by excess fluid), and this information may guide the surgeon's method of treatment. In addition, many of the specialized refractive surgeries involving the cornea require that the corneal thickness be known in order to make proper decisions in planning for and performing the surgery.

Corneal thickness pachymetry is just another form of A-scan biometry. Usually the instruments used do not have a display screen to observe as do the axial length units, but they are A-scans nonetheless.

The root word "pachy" means thickness and "meter" refers to a measuring device. Therefore, a pachymeter is an instrument for measuring thickness. Recently, a new word has been coined that means the same thing as pachymetry.

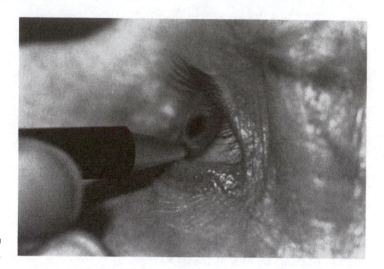

Figure 2.3 A tiny transducer is gently placed against the anesthetized cornea to obtain a corneal thickness measurement.

The new word is "pachometry" and does occasionally show up in printed texts. Personally, I prefer the word pachymetry as it is more accurately based on the word roots, but you should expect to see either one used.

DIAGNOSTIC B-SCAN

As touched upon in the first chapter, the B-scan is a two-dimensional imaging technique that reveals the geometry and geography of ocular structures. The size, shape, and location of anatomical features can be easily determined using this examination method.

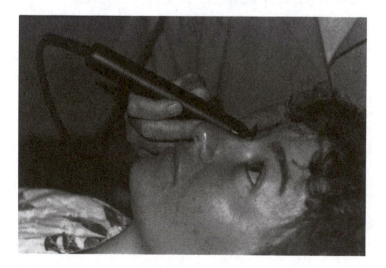

Figure 2.4 In the open eye B-scan technique, the probe is placed on the anesthetized sclera. A series of probe movements allows the examiner to examine all aspects of the globe and orbit.

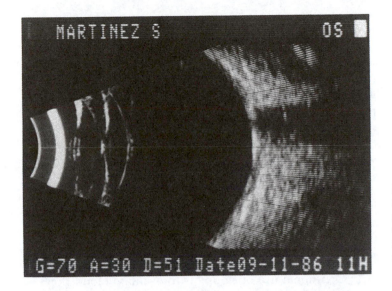

Figure 2.5 The classic normal B-scan echogram from a patient's left eye displays echoes from both corneal surfaces, both lens surfaces, retina, optic nerve, and orbital fat.

What are the indications for performing a diagnostic B-scan? Quite simply, any time there is an opaque medium through which the surgeon cannot evaluate the condition of the posterior segment of the globe, or if there is an indication of an orbital pathology such as proptosis or the protrusion of an eye from the socket, a B-scan is indicated.

A simple way of thinking about this is also useful as a way of explaining to the patient the need for this test: "If you can't see out of that eye, the doctor can't see in. The sound waves will make a picture of the inside of your eye

The most common indication for performing a diagnostic B-scan is an opaque media— that is, when a clear view into the eye cannot be obtained with more simple devices, such as a slit lamp or retinoscope.

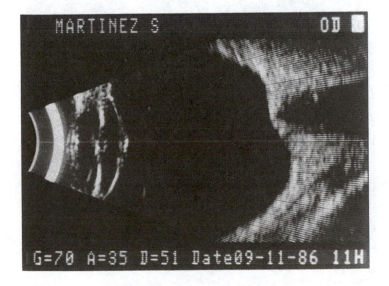

Figure 2.6 The same patient's right eye, however, displays a very different curvature of the globe. This unusual staphyloma (irregularly shaped globe) shows multiple curvatures of the posterior aspect.

so that we can evaluate the parts which cannot be examined by shining a light into the eye."

There are two schools of thought concerning the ultimate value of B-scan information. One group feels confident that through experience, very positive diagnoses may be made with the B-scan alone, or with the B-scan and its accompanying A-scan. Since a B-scan is made up of a sum of A-scans, most instruments permit any one of the B-scan lines to be pulled out of the image and displayed below the B-scan. This is called a cross-vector A-scan.

The other school of thought believes that the B-scan, even with a cross-vector A-scan, does not provide enough information and that the final diagnosis in most situations should be made with a combination of tools:

1. Standardized, diagnostic A-scan
2. Contact B-scan
3. Occasional use of doppler (to evaluate blood flow)

Another indication for B-scan is proptosis. When one eye appears to be displaced from its normal position, there could be a problem in the orbit or with the eye's muscles. B-scan is an especially useful and cost-effective method for examining extraocular structures as well as intraocular ones.

This multiple technique will be discussed in chapter 7.

The overall shape of the globe, the insertion and separation points of a membrane, the position of a foreign body with respect to an anatomical structure, and the size and extent of a tumor are all easily determined with B-scans. They can also be quite useful in making dynamic evaluations. This involves observing the after movement or lack of after movement of structures as they relate to natural eye movements.

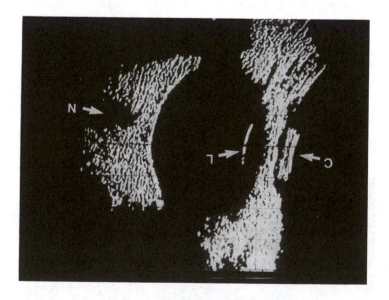

Figure 2.7 The water bath or immersion B-scan produces slightly different images than the contact scanners. There are fewer gray tones in this scan, producing a crisp image.

One such type of dynamic evaluation would be to observe the "wriggle" of an unknown membrane in the eye. A quick, fluid movement could indicate that the membrane in question is a vitreous detachment, whereas a more stiff, subdued movement may lead the examiner to suspect a retinal detachment instead.

This type of dynamic evaluation may seem largely subjective. However, the practice of scanning eyes for which the diagnosis has already been made assists with the communication of these observations in a less subjective manner.

Dynamic evaluations of echoes are made during the exam, not afterward. The subtle movements of structures can give an experienced echographer an extra puzzle piece needed to assist in making a diagnosis.

The B-scan is sometimes called contact B-scan. That refers to using the B-scan probe directly on the surface of the eye. This can be on the closed lid or directly on the anesthetized sclera or cornea. There is one other type of B-scan, however. It is called water bath or immersion B-scan. The equipment for performing this type of scan is no longer manufactured, but is still used in a few locations. It involves gluing a waterproof drape around the eye of a supine patient. The top of the drape is held in a ring stand. A lid speculum is inserted in the eye and about one liter of sterile saline is poured into the drape.

At this time, a mechanical apparatus holding a transducer is lowered so that it is submerged in the saline. The crystal is then moved back and forth by hand using a small lever. This type of scanning can produce good images, but is time consuming and not very comfortable for the patient. Modern contact B-scanning equipment is capable of producing exceptionally clear, high-resolution images in a more "user friendly" and "patient friendly" manner.

STANDARDIZED ECHOGRAPHY

As mentioned above, standardized echography is a form of ophthalmic echography which utilizes primarily two forms of diagnostic ultrasound with the occasional use of doppler. The two forms of diagnostic scanning are standardized diagnostic A-scan and contact B-scan. In addition to utilizing these two modes, there is one more important aspect of this technique, and that is the use of standardized examination procedures. This method has been developed over the last two and a half decades. In the beginning, only A-scan was available and later B-scan was incorporated into the technique.

Karl C. Ossoinig, MD, is the pioneer in this field, having

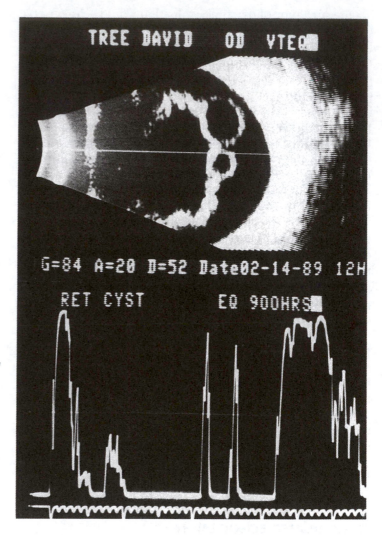

Figure 2.8 *Standardized echography is a combination of methods and techniques. This B-scan of a long-standing retinal detachment shows retinal cysts which are fluid-filled. The corresponding standardized A-scan shows two echoes, one each from the front and back of the larger cyst. The lack of echoes between these spikes indicates that the lesion is fluid-filled.*

Standardized echography is a fascinating subspecialty in the field of diagnostic ultrasound. Trained echographers can readily identify most common ocular disorders and many not-so-common ones as well by using a combination of methods.

developed the equipment and techniques and the clinical data base that is critically important in the teaching of others.

With the application of standardized echography techniques, both the globe and orbit are carefully and systematically scanned. This allows the examiner to be certain that all areas have been thoroughly assessed. This method does however require equipment with unusually precise characteristics. In addition to specialized equipment, a formal course of study and preferably a certain amount of on-location training is desirable. This will be discussed further in chapter 7.

CONCLUDING REMARKS

In summary, it is helpful to understand the various ways in which ultrasound is used in ophthalmology. It may not be necessary or appropriate for every technician to be able to perform all types of examinations. However, the knowledge of which methods will provide the clinical information needed to properly diagnose each patient could make a difference in the management of that patient.

It is always correct to ask for help or a second opinion. For example, it may be appropriate to refer a cataract patient for a B-scan when an abnormal axial length is measured. This could postpone a planned surgery until the integrity of the retina is confirmed. Knowledge of how to best help the patient is the ultimate goal of any diagnostic procedure.

It is always correct to request assistance or a second opinion. Even the most experienced examiners will call one another and discuss an echographic finding. We learn best when we share our experiences with others.

CHAPTER 3

Instrumentation

SIMILAR COMPONENTS

Although no two models of ophthalmic ultrasound instrumentation are exactly alike, there are some fundamental similarities. To begin with, let's look at the most basic design of an ultrasound unit.

Each unit will have a console of some type. The console is indicated by the heavy black rectangle in Figure 3.1. It is here that the probe is activated and where sound waves from ocular structures are processed for display.

The features that perform the same functions in all devices are:

1. Probe or probes
2. Pulse emitter
3. Receiver
4. Amplifier
5. Signal processor
6. Display
7. Image documentation

Although no two instruments look alike, even when they are made by the same manufacturer, all ultrasound units have many similar components and work in the same fundamental way.

Probes

Each ultrasound unit will have at least one probe. There are four different examination methods, each of which has its own probe. These are:

1. Axial eye length biometry A-scan
2. Standardized and nonstandardized diagnostic A-scan
3. Corneal thickness pachymetry A-scan
4. Diagnostic B-scan

Axial Length A-scan

The probe for performing contact axial eye length scans is available as solid-tipped, or with a water bath or nose cone attached. The hollow nose cone has a thin membrane placed

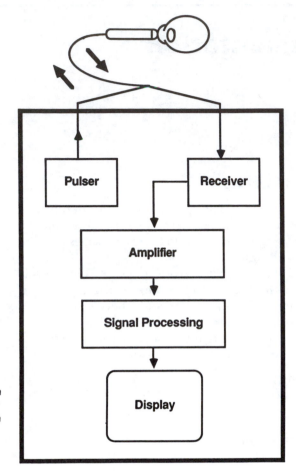

Figure 3.1 The fundamental components of any ultrasound device are a pulse emitter that sends electricity to the probe, a receiver to "hear" the echoes, an amplifier to enlarge them, a signal processor for reshaping, and a display for viewing the images.

over the tip. Distilled water is then injected inside. Usually there is an internal fixation light in a contact probe to assist the patient during the exam. The frequency of these probes is between 10 and 12 MHz.

Diagnostic A-scan

A diagnostic A-scan probe is different from a biometry probe. It may be either standardized or nonstandardized. Standardized A-scan probes are always solid-tipped and have the same frequency and beam shape. Nonstandardized diagnostic A-scan probes are usually solid. Some equipment manufacturers may utilize their axial length biometry probes for diagnostic scanning. The probe designed specifically for standardized diagnostic A-scan does not have an internal fixation light and its frequency is 8 MHz.

Corneal Thickness A-scan

The probe for performing corneal thickness pachymetry is smaller than the axial length probe. Also, the frequency is higher since more resolution is required for measuring such a small structure. There is no fixation light in this probe and the frequency can be 12 to 15 MHz.

Since A-scan probes have no moving parts, they are smaller than B-scan probes. Both may be of the permanently sealed or solid type, or may have to be disassembled and cleaned.

Diagnostic B-scan

An ultrasound unit may also have a B-scan probe. This will always be a bit larger than an A-scan probe because it has moving parts. Inside a fluid-filled chamber, a crystal oscillates sending sound waves out in a fan-like array called a sector scan or polar scan. This sector creates the well-known fan shape of an ophthalmic B-scan display.

The B-scan probe does not have a built-in fixation light and the frequency is 10 MHz. There may be probes available with different frequencies for special applications. A higher frequency of 12 MHz may be useful for examining the anterior segment, while an orbital surgeon would prefer a lower frequency such as 7 MHz for imaging deeper structures.

Transducer

There is one part common to all ultrasound probes, and that is the transducer. As explained in the first chapter, the transducer in the application of ultrasound is a special crystal capable of transforming electrical energy into mechanical energy (in the form of a sound wave). Conversely, it converts sound energy into electrical energy that may be processed and displayed on a screen.

Pulse Emitter

The pulse emitter is the part of the unit responsible for providing an electrical signal that the transducer converts into sound waves.

Often the emitter is called a pulse emitter because the

electricity is sent to the crystal in pulses, somewhat like a strobe light. A strobe light does not produce an even source of light, rather it turns on and off very rapidly. A similar effect is necessary in the operation of ophthalmic ultrasound systems because there is only one crystal inside each probe to send and receive the sound waves. The reason we use only one crystal to share both jobs is to ensure that the size of the probes will be kept to a minimum.

Receiver

During the brief period when the emitter is not producing electrical energy, the receiver is receiving the signals the transducer has "heard." The sound waves reflected directly back to the crystal are converted by the transducer into electrical signals. The job of the receiver is to collect these signals and send them on to the amplifier.

Amplifier

The amplifier simply enlarges or amplifies the returning echo signal. This larger echo may be more readily sculpted at the next destination, the signal processor.

Signal Processor

The art of designing an ultrasound system lies in the field of signal processing. Creating a system that will detect tiny echoes from the eye while filtering out noise is the goal of each design engineer. Obviously, some do a better job than others, so it is important to compare systems with clinical evaluation of pathologies, not simply normal eyes.

The field of signal processing is where design engineers show us their artistic creativity. The quality and type of echo that will appear on the screen is in large measure controlled by this part of the system. The different methods of processing the signals are evidenced by the fact that the images produced by devices from different manufacturers are so varied. Some engineers prefer the smooth, rounded appearance created by an analog display, while others prefer the squared-off look of digital signal processors.

The examiner should choose a system that will allow him or her to best utilize the methods by which they perform examinations. When shopping for an ultrasound system, it is important to try out several different kinds so that an educated evaluation may be made. This will benefit all involved—the technician, the physician, and the patient. Features of one ultrasound unit that are a requirement for one echographer may be useless for another.

Display Screen

The majority of units have a built-in viewing screen in the console for actively observing the ultrasound images representative of ocular tissues. It is my opinion that having a clearly viewed screen at all times is mandatory. I cannot support the idea of performing any type of ultrasound scan on an eye and accepting a readout for which there is no visible scan. My training plus my experience with the behavior of electronic instruments tells me that my interpretation of the scan is the final say on whether or not the readout is acceptable. Therefore, in this book it will be assumed that the phrase "ultrasound unit" refers to an instrument which has a display screen.

Observing the echograms on a display screen is mandatory while making axial length measurements. It is important to visually verify the integrity of each of the A-scan echoes prior to accepting the results produced by the instrument.

Measuring Gates

Most units will have some way of indicating which portion of the scan is being measured. In an A-scan, these measurement markers are usually called gates, calipers, or overlights. In the B-scan, they are more often referred to as just calipers.

A-scan Gates

There are a variety of ways that manufacturers may choose to display a measuring gate. Some are located underneath the echoes near the base line while others actually trace the entire outline of the echo. Still others have a vertical line which is positioned to the left of the echo being measured, and there is yet another type of unit that has a threshold line that changes in elevation or brightness when in contact with the echo being measured. All perform exactly the same function: somehow we must have a way of telling the instrument which of the echoes are to be used to determine the axial length, lens thickness, chamber depth, muscle thickness, tumor height, or any other selected feature.

B-scan Calipers

It is not known who first began using the term caliper for measuring a structure on a B-scan, but it is widely used today. On a B-scan, the desired measurement may be of the base of a tumor, for example, which is a vertical dimension on the screen. The height of the tumor, from front to back, is also a very useful parameter. Both are used to document the growth of shrinkage of a tumor. Two small crosses are the most common appearance of a B-scan caliper.

The accuracy of measurements varies not only from unit to unit, but in general the left/right (horizontal) measurements will be more accurate than the up/down (vertical) ones. This has to do with other principles that are not necessarily important to cover at this time. What is important is that you know the tolerances and abilities of the instrument being used.

Tolerance is the range in which a measurement may occur. For example, accuracy may be rated as plus or minus 0.15 mm. This means that if the readout on the display says 10 mm, it could really be anywhere from 9.85 mm to 10.15 mm. The term tolerance is frequently used and should be taken into consideration when working with the measured values.

Image Documentation Devices

It is one thing to see a scan on the screen and make an evaluation of it, and quite another thing to explain what you saw to someone else. That is where the practice of documenting images comes into play. There are basically two types of images to document, stationary and moving. The ultrasound images may be saved by five different methods:

1. Polaroid photographs
2. 35 mm photographs
3. Ink prints
4. Thermal prints
5. Videotapes

There is a wide range of devices that document images. Experiment with different films, printers, etc. Choose one or more that not only suit your needs but provide stable images for future reference.

Polaroid Photographs

The most common method of documenting either an A-scan or a B-scan is to simply take a picture of it. Generally, this is done with a Polaroid camera often mounted to the unit with a hinge mechanism. The camera is positioned in front of the display screen and the shutter is depressed when the desired image appears on the screen.

The type of film used will depend upon two things, the camera style and whether the image is frozen or active. The major advantage of taking a Polaroid photograph is having immediate feedback about the quality of the preserved image. In this way, if the photo is not good enough, another picture may be taken before the patient leaves the office.

35 mm Photographs

Some clinics prefer the cost effectiveness of 35 mm film and will have this type of camera mounted in some manner on the console. The disadvantage of this technique is that most of the time the film is not developed until after the patient has left. This of course makes it very difficult to recreate the images in the event that the pictures don't turn out. 35 mm photography is generally reserved for the more experienced photographer.

Polapan is a type of black and white 35 mm slide film manufactured by Polaroid that is quite appropriate for ultrasound use. What makes it especially nice is that with a small table top unit about the size of a shoe box the film may be developed in a matter of minutes. After developing, the pictures can be inspected to be certain the images are of good quality before sending the patient home. The slides may be mounted.

Ink Prints

Some systems have either a built-in or separate ink printer that will produce a copy of the image shown on the screen. This type of printer is only adequate for documenting axial length scans. It is a very durable print that will maintain the image for a very long time.

Thermal Prints

Thermal printers generate an image using a process whereby heat-sensitive paper is contacted with a hot needle and a black mark is produced. Thermal printers may be used for both A-scan and B-scan images. When a print of this type is made of a B-scan, it is done with a separate video printer rather than a built-in printer.

It is important to know that thermal paper can seriously degrade over a period of time. Therefore, it is common practice that the most important thermal images to be saved for the patient's chart are photocopied to assure image stability. New advances are being made every year in the quality of thermal paper, however. Perhaps manufacturers will soon develop a method of preventing the images from fading. In the meantime, it is recommended that for medical and legal reasons, critical images made by a thermal process be photocopied.

Videotapes

In order to document a moving image, video equipment is required. If the ultrasound unit has a jack (connector) on the back panel labeled "video out," the only equipment required is a video cassette recorder (VCR) and a monitor for viewing the tapes after they are made. Some units will allow the videotapes to be played back through the same screen that is used for viewing the original scans. Other units require that a video camera be used in place of the Polaroid, or that a scan converter be used to convert the image to one that a VCR can easily record.

When making videotapes, add a simultaneous audio recording explaining probe position or have some method of marking the tape with probe orientation data. This is essential information for making a complete diagnosis.

There are a few less desirable aspects of videotaping an examination. One has to do with the difficulty of labeling tapes as to the orientation of the B-scan probe with respect to the eye. Since this is the only way of knowing where in the eye or orbit a pathology is located, it is of utmost importance to properly document an examination. If the unit is equipped with a probe position indicator, attention must be paid to continuously monitoring this marker.

When playing back the video recording, it is sometimes seen that although the scans were good, the examiner neglected to move the indicator or put labels on the screen to show the orientation of the probe. Without proper labeling, these ultrasound images may be beautiful to look at, but clinically they are practically useless. Since the eye is basically round, B-scans from entirely different locations in the eye may appear identical on the screen. It is only the examiner's markings that tell the whole story.

Another consideration in videotaping is the fact that a scrupulously accurate log must be kept, noting the date, patient name and counter number from the video recorder. When it comes time to look up a patient's images, it can be time consuming and frustrating to search for a few minutes' worth of images on a two-hour tape if good records are not kept. Finally, proper storage of tapes is important in order to assure both their ability to play without sticking or jamming and to maintain image quality.

ANALOG VERSUS DIGITAL

In order to better understand the similarities and differences between specific instruments, we must first clarify one more issue, analog versus digital displays. Generally speaking, the older types of equipment are analog and the newer ones are digital, but of course there are always exceptions. There are fundamental operating characteristics that are different between the two types. In the following chapters where the particular techniques of performing scans are discussed, reference will be made to the type of technique used.

One obvious difference in the operation of the machines is simply that the digital unit permits the technician to freeze the scan by means of a foot pedal, whereas in an analog unit the image is always moving. There are also some hybrid systems available whereby the image appears in an analog format yet it can be frozen.

In terms of the actual image, there are differences as well. One apt analogy is that an analog image is like a drawing of a rose, with curved lines that may be made exactly as the artist wishes. On the other hand, a digital image is like a needlepoint of a rose; there can be no curved lines, but with many stitches made in the checkerboard pattern the contours almost look round. In fact, the more stitches per inch that are made, the more round it appears.

An analog image is like a drawing of a rose made with curves and angled lines. A digital image is like needlepoint artwork, having many small steps, or "stitches" that make up the picture.

Analog Equipment

In a fully analog system, the image continually moves and the examiner must evaluate the image while the probe is in contact with the eye. Also, each photograph must be taken while peeking through a viewing door on the top of the camera—one hand poised on the shutter switch while the other holds the probe in just the right position on the eye. There are times when this can be quite a juggling act.

The analog image has a more realistic look. This is especially noticeable in the A-mode. When you look closely at the A-scan echoes from an analog image, you will see that the edges are smooth and not made up of step-like increments. An analog screen is capable of producing both angled and curved lines. This can be particularly useful when interpreting information from individual A-scan echoes and will be discussed further in chapter 4. It should be pointed out that an analog display is required when performing a standardized diagnostic A-scan.

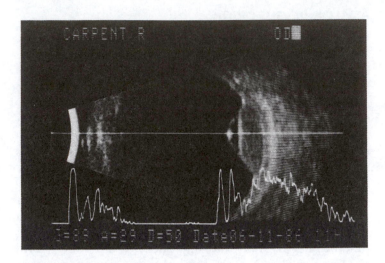

Figure 3.2 This analog image of a choroidal melanoma with an elevated retinal detachment over it, shows smooth echoes on the cross vector A-scan displayed below. The first tall echo under the tumor is from the retina, the second is from the tumor surface.

Digital Equipment

In the digital representation of an A-scan, the stair step or squared off appearance is easily seen on every echo. Why go to the digital format then, if the analog format provides such attractive images? The main reason is to obtain a video output signal for making videotapes and video prints. Although it is possible to have an analog system with freeze frame, these units cannot have direct video outputs.

The squared-off type of digital display is also noticeable on a B-scan image and it is a matter of becoming accustomed to the type of system being used so that correct interpretations may be made.

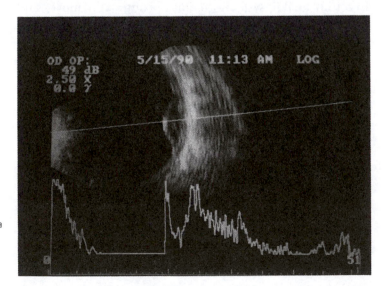

Figure 3.3 This digital image of another choroidal melanoma shows the "stair steps" on the cross vector A-scan image that are created by the digitization of the scan.

In a digital unit, the examiner presses a foot switch and freezes the image on the screen for additional evaluation and measurement while the patient is allowed to rest. The frozen image may be altered in its appearance by applying a variety of postprocessing functions. If the frozen image is to be documented after inspection, the camera is positioned in front of the screen and a picture is taken. Also, if a VCR is available, a recording of the real time scan as it is happening may be made in addition to a still photo of any frozen scan.

A Little of Both

As mentioned above, there is also the possibility that an ultrasound instrument may have a little of both analog and digital imaging characteristics. The echoes may be smooth as in an analog image, yet still have the ability to be frozen like a digital unit. This is accomplished with a digital memory circuit that enables the unit to memorize one scan at a time. In this type of unit, hookup to a VCR is possible with the use of a scan converter, or a standard video camera may photograph the screen. Since use of video recordings of B-scan examinations is not that common, many feel that they would rather have what they consider to be improvements in image quality rather than direct video and postprocessing features.

In the future, digital units will use higher resolution, more expensive monitors and electronics that will allow the images to more closely resemble those of the analog display format. But as the needlepoint analogy illustrates, there will always be differences in the image. There have been enormous improvements in the quality of all ultrasound instrumentation over the past several years, and there is no reason to think that the development is slowing. As long as there are technicians, physicians, and echographers who keep asking for more and better functions in their equipment, there will be companies with clever engineers ready to try and fill their needs.

TROUBLESHOOTING

Many service calls to manufacturers are made when there are no real problems with the equipment. Therefore, when something goes wrong, try to devote only the first few seconds to total panic. Then take all of the energy used in being upset and apply it to the situation at hand. Easier

When an equipment failure is experienced, go into a panic for no more than a few seconds. Then put all that energy to work tracing the pathways of the instrument before calling for help. Many service problems may be solved by clear thinking and perseverance on the part of the operator.

said than done, right? Depending on the nature of the problem, begin at the point where the probe comes in contact with the patient and trace the pathway all the way back to the wall outlet where the unit is plugged in. Somewhere along that pathway there may be an easily detectable fault causing your examination to come to a halt.

Let's look at each of the major components of an ultrasound device for clues about where to look for operator solvable problems. If, after trying these solutions the equipment is still not functioning properly, by all means call the service department.

Probes

Probes are probably the main culprit when it comes to downtime. Careful handling, cleaning, and frequent inspection can minimize problems. As discussed in the first chapter, the crystal inside the probe is the heart of any ultrasound unit. Since it has a voltage applied to it constantly, it is likely to lose its sensitivity over time. This can happen quickly or slowly.

When a transducer loses its sensitivity slowly, what is noticed is that the gain must be increased in order to obtain the same echo height (A-scan) or brightness (B-scan) on the screen. This can occur even with the most conscientious care. It is impossible to predict the lifetime of any probe—some last only months, others last years. The following discussion of individual probe types may provide ideas that will ensure the longest possible transducer life.

There are two things that all probes have in common, the ceramic plate transducer and the connector or plug. With all the attention to caring for the probe tip, don't neglect the other end. Every time a probe is connected to or removed from a console, be gentle. Realize that inside that strong-appearing connector there are many tiny, delicate wires. If even one wire gets broken, the effect will be quite noticeable to the operator.

A broken wire in the probe's connector may cause the probe to go completely dead and give no echo information at all or it can cause the echoes to jump up and down on the screen, owing to an intermittent connection. It may also cause a "noisy" echogram having many small echoes that get in the way of interpreting the scan. Once this is noticed, the probe should immediately be returned to the manufacturer for repair before more damage occurs.

When possible, send the service department a photograph depicting the problem. Remember, a picture is worth a thousand words, and often the people performing the service are not clinicians and may not really understand your description of the problem.

Water-filled A-scan Probes

Most manufactures provide a syringe with a blunt needle for filling the probe. Don't substitute a regular sharp needle for two reasons: (1) the sharp needle can and often does cause damage by scratching the surface of the crystal, and (2) the small diameter of the sharp needle may cause excess agitation of the water thereby increasing the possibility of introducing microscopic air bubbles. These tiny bubbles will inevitably prevent the ultrasound energy from being properly transmitted through the eye.

For a probe filled with distilled water, the single most common problem is that of air bubbles inside the probe. These can produce incorrect measurements and can create strange echo patterns on the screen even before making contact with the eye.

There are two effective methods of removing air bubbles. The first is to remove some of the water with the syringe, creating a large air pocket in the probe. Next, tilt and turn the probe so that the large bubble comes into contact with the smaller ones. Once they are all collected together, inject water in a slow yet steady flow until the air is pushed out.

The second method is to add a very small amount of contact lens wetting solution to the distilled water so that the bubbles become slippery. They will be less likely to stick to the inside of the probe and will be more easily pushed out of the filling hole as water is injected. Be careful not to add too much wetting solution because it can create foam, making matters worse. One drop per probe is sufficient.

Even with a properly filled probe, there will always be two and often three echoes on the screen. The first is from the surface of the crystal and the second is from the membrane on the tip of the nose cone. Occasionally, a third echo occurs that is a reverberation from the membrane echo. This third echo, if present, is substantially reduced or disappears when the probe contacts the cornea. Becoming accustomed to the pattern for a particular probe and instrument will help alert the operator to a potential problem if an abnormal pattern appears prior to or during the scan. The probe tip membranes are easily torn and must be frequently inspected.

Solid-tipped A-scan Probes

Although there are usually fewer problems with the solid probes, damage to the crystal can occur if the probe is dropped or the wire is accidentally pulled out. Always check the condition of the tip for nicks or sharp edges if the probe is accidentally dropped.

Internal Fixation Light

Nowadays, most axial eye length probes come equipped with a built-in fixation light to assist the patient in looking straight ahead. For some probes, the light is a function independent of the ceramic plate sending out the sound energy. Therefore, if the light is not working, don't panic yet, for the transducer may still operate properly. Check the transducer function by putting a drop of saline solution on the probe tip and observe the screen for a series of jiggling echoes. If the probe is sending out sound energy, you can still use it—simply provide a fellow eye fixation target. You can call the service department later after the patient's scans have been completed.

B-scan Probes

In any ultrasound unit, there are only two moving parts, the cooling fan and the crystal inside the B-scan probe. As you might guess, the cooling fan rarely if ever breaks. The B-scan probe is rather a different story. When there are delicate moving parts, there are more likely to be break-downs, especially when the human hand comes into contact with the parts. The B-scan probe is apt to fail if dropped. For those who have one that requires filling with distilled water, this must never be done when the probe is operating. The blunt needle rule, as discussed above, applies here as well. Never substitute a sharp needle because damage to the crystal could occur. In addition, storing the probe dry when not used for extended periods is always a good idea.

For the so-called permanently filled probes, there is still a need to check for air bubbles since some probes will develop them over a period of time. Air bubbles in the probe will of course affect the image by causing artifacts (unwanted echoes) or if the bubble is large enough, part or all of the image may be missing.

Keep all probes cleaned of fluids and gel. Keep dust covers on when instruments are not in use. Know where the instruction manual is kept.

If the oil or other fluid that fills a sealed probe is observed on the outside of the probe body, check for holes in the membrane and cracks in the body. Do not use a leaky probe on a patient, especially in an open eye technique. The fluid inside the probe is definitely not a sterile ophthalmic solution and could cause irritation. Contact the service department immediately before any further damage occurs.

Polaroid Camera

There are two kinds of Polaroid cameras used in ophthalmic echography. These are a manual type and an automatic type. In the manual camera, type 667 film is used for analog units without freeze frame. Type 611 film is used in manual cameras for units with freeze frame. In the manual camera, the single most common problem is jamming of the film when it is pulled out of the camera by the operator. This could be caused by several things. First, the operator may not be pulling the film out in a straight, slow, and uniform manner. Secondly, the rollers inside the film door very often have a buildup of developing chemicals. These rollers should be examined every time a new pack of film is loaded, and removed and cleaned whenever the slightest buildup is noticed. They can be cleaned by rinsing the rollers in hot running tap water or by scrubbing with an alcohol prep pad. Be certain the rollers are completely dry before returning them to the camera. Thirdly, film jams will also occur in manual cameras when the small white tabs in the film pack get caught in the film door as it is being closed after a new pack has been loaded. To prevent this, hold the tabs back while closing the film door.

The automatic cameras, or auto-backs as they are often called, have their own set of problems. Even though the film is automatically ejected from the pack, thereby reducing the incidence of jammed film, this problem still occurs. The number one cause of jammed film, or film that does not come out all the way, is failure of the power source for the mechanism which ejects the film. This power is supplied either by batteries in a pack attached to the camera or by a wire that attaches the camera to the console or electrical outlet.

In the case of a battery-powered camera, there are two points worth mentioning. First of all, it really does pay to buy good quality batteries. Gold-topped ones from Kodak or copper-topped ones from Duracell are substantially bet-

Use only top-notch batteries in cameras. The gold- and copper-topped ones really are superior to the no-name brands It's worth the few extra pennies spent to ensure a properly working camera.

ter than other types. The motor requires quite a bit of power and will misbehave when cheap batteries get even a little low on energy. In addition, you would be surprised to learn how many cameras are returned to service departments as defective when the real problem is that someone put the batteries in backward. Take the time to check out the drawings that are usually on the inside of the battery pack, or ask someone's help if you are not sure how the batteries fit.

In the case of a camera which receives its power from the ultrasound console, remember that there are two points of connection that have to be secure in order for the current to get from the unit to the camera. These two points are the plug that goes into the unit and the plug that goes into the camera. If the camera is not operating properly, unplug each of these connectors, inspect them and reinsert the plugs to be certain that they are making good contact. If that doesn't solve the problem, call the service department and ask for a new camera cable before assuming that the camera needs replacing.

When the cause of film jamming cannot be located in the batteries or power supply, it could be the result of a bad pack of film or a defect in the mechanism that ejects the film. Try a new pack of film first. In the case of blurred photos, be sure that the camera is held still while the shutter is open. If the images seem washed out and dim, check the exposure time on the camera. Images that are too bright may require less exposure time; dim ones need more exposure time.

Display Screen

The problem of a washed-out or dim image may be visible on the screen as well as on the photos. If so, check the rear panel controls for the screen contrast and brightness. A few experimental photos at different camera and equipment settings will help to determine the optimum values. If the problem is the lack of any display on the screen, a number of factors could be involved. It could be as simple as the image position knobs (up/down and right/left) being in the wrong position so that the scan was inadvertently shifted off the screen. Moving these controls might result in locating the image.

Another thing to try is to make sure that the type of scan that is to be performed has been selected on the unit, either by pushing a button or turning a knob to a specific position.

If some information other than the ultrasound image is seen on the screen, but not the actual A- or B-scan, the problem usually lies with the probe. Of course, the lack of an image could simply be the result of a probe that is not plugged in all the way, and therefore not making a good electrical connection. And don't forget to inspect the probe for air bubbles.

If all of these suggestions don't help, then maybe there really is something wrong with the probe or console. It is always a good idea to try another probe with the unit if one is available to see if it will produce an image. This will show if it is the probe or the unit that is not working.

Often with systems that are menu driven or operate similarly to a computer, a glitch may occur which produces strange behavior or an inability of the instrument to advance or retreat in the program. When in doubt, simply turn the unit off, count to three, and turn it back on. With a computer driven instrument, it is not advisable to turn it off and on too quickly. Switching it back on too soon can sometimes scramble its thinking, causing a worse problem than the one you were trying to correct.

There is one more thing to be aware of when evaluating problems on the screen. It is quite normal for electrical "noise" to be present in the images when a laser is operating in close proximity to an ultrasound device. Ultrasound is very susceptible to interference when such high voltage equipment is being used nearby. The noise can look like fuzz, or grass on the base line of an A-scan, or tiny glints or flashes of light scattered throughout the B-scan image. To verify the source of the noise on the image, try turning off different pieces of equipment and then observing the quality of the image.

If there are no nearby instruments turned on that could account for the noise on the image, try gently, very gently wiggling the wires of the probes. First move the wires where they connect to the machine, then where they connect to the probe, while observing the screen for any change in the appearance of the image. If an improvement or a worsening of the image is noted, contact the service department and report a poor electrical connection in the probe. If the problem exists where the probe plugs into the unit, which is more likely the case since this is the part that comes into contact with the hand most frequently, then it can probably be easily repaired. When the poor connection is inside the probe, it can be much more difficult to repair. Consult with the manufacturer for their recommendations.

Foot Switch and Power

When the unit will not turn on, or when the foot switch doesn't work right or work at all, check to see that the connectors are plugged in correctly. Even if they look plugged in, unplug them anyway and then reconnect them to the unit. The next thing to look for is a bent, broken, or missing pin in the connector. When cables are not plugged in carefully, the pins can be damaged resulting in a poor connection. One additional possibility is that there may be something wrong with the outlet into which the machine is plugged. Check to see that the receptacle is good by trying a lamp or other known working item, or take the ultrasound unit to a different room to see if it works there.

Fuses

If the power cord is plugged in properly and the outlet in the wall is working, but still the unit seems dead, then by all means check its fuses. Usually they are located on the rear panel of the console near the power cord. Know where these are, have the properly rated spares on hand and know how to change them. It is amazingly simple, and once you have done it, you will never forget. If you don't know where they are or how to change them, call the service department and ask a technician to guide you through the process over the phone.

Calling for Service

A time may arrive when you have tried everything and still there is a problem with the equipment. OK, it's time to call the service department. When calling, be prepared with as much information as possible for the service technician. Be sure to have the model and serial number of the equipment handy. Take a photo of any questionable images to send along with the instrument should it need to be returned to the factory. Always keep the phone numbers of the company headquarters and local representatives with the unit. Remember to take into consideration the difference in time zones between where you are and where the service department is. This will help to reduce frustration and unanswered calls. Also, if you are currently working with a patient, try not to let them know too much about the problem so that they will not become unduly concerned.

There is nothing more frustrating to a service technician than the complaint "My machine is not working!" Now think about it. How would you respond to a patient who called in and said, "My eye has something wrong with it"? You would have to immediately start asking questions: Is there pain, redness, itching, blurred or lost vision, or flashes of light? So don't be surprised if the technician on the other end of the telephone asks similar questions of you. Try to mentally note or write down the symptoms as best as you can so that the service people will be given as much information as possible and an efficient course of action may be taken. Also remember that service personnel often are not familiar with clinical details, and since you both speak different technical languages it will require some mutual patience.

Find out before you have equipment problems what the manufacturer's policies are regarding warranties, service and loaners. Get all guarantees in writing to avoid aggravation later when no one remembers what promises were made.

When returning an instrument to the factory for service it is best to use the original packaging materials. Most equipment is shipped to the customer with custom foam inserts and a box large enough to provide several inches of space between the unit and the box. If the unit is not packed properly, shipping damage will inevitably occur. I have seen a several-thousand-dollar B-scan probe returned in a Federal Express overnight envelope! Also, one office returned a 45-pound instrument wrapped in a table cloth and placed in a large diaper box. Needless to say, the unit was nearly destroyed by the shipping. Ask the service department for packaging advice.

Loaner Equipment

Some companies offer to send out loaner probes to use while yours is being repaired. The policy of one company may differ significantly from another, so be sure to get any such guarantees in writing. Failure to do so may cause problems long after the unit has been purchased and the original salesperson is not available to confirm the fact that you were promised something.

Loaner equipment is very expensive for companies to maintain because of the additional shipping costs, the damage to loaned equipment, and the incredibly difficult time they have in getting loaner pieces back from customers. Once an original probe has been repaired and returned, many customers do not have a compelling reason to return the loaner in an expedient manner. Some people even wait until the company asks for it to be returned, hoping they will forget that it was loaned. This makes the availability of loaners even more scarce.

Service Contracts

Some companies offer maintenance agreements or service contracts extending the original warranty on the equipment. There are several factors to be evaluated when buying such a contract. Be very clear about exactly what is included in the contract. Some contracts cover the console and all the accessories while others cover the console only and not the B-probe or the camera. Take into consideration the cost of repairing or replacing any items not covered in the contract when weighing the overall costs of maintaining your equipment.

The price of a service contact will, of course, vary from one company to another, and from one product to another. A general rule which may be applied, however, is to estimate the service contract's annual cost at ten percent of the purchase price. Therefore, if an ultrasound system costs $25,000 for example, the service contract could cost $2,500 per year. It is not unusual for the price to go up, the older the system becomes, for obviously an older system is more likely to experience a failure.

CLEANING THE CONSOLE

There are a number of areas to maintain on the ultrasound console. First of all, be sure to keep the knobs clean. Usually a damp cloth or in most cases an alcohol prep pad may be used to clean dried coupling gel from the knobs and front panel. If you are unsure whether or not alcohol may be used, consult the instruction manual or call the customer service department.

In the same way, the probe holder must be kept spotlessly clean. Remember that if a used probe (one with gel still on the tip after having examined a patient) is put back into the probe holder, then the holder will be contaminated. When the probes are cleaned after each patient, follow through by cleaning the probe holders at the same time.

One final part of the console to pay attention to is the exhaust fan. Often the fan's filter becomes clogged with dust. The good news is that the dirt did not get into the console. The bad news is that the dirtier the fan filter, the less able the fan will be to do the job of keeping the unit cool. Poor cooling will shorten the lifetime of components inside the instrument.

Vacuuming is one of the best ways to clean the filter. A can of compressed air used for dusting negatives may also be used, but realize that if the dust is sent back into the air, it will probably end up on the filter again. Maintaining proper ventilation is the most important thing you can do to take care of the console.

AN EXPERIMENT

When I was in college, my electronics professor conducted a lab experiment which proved to be quite instructive to we students who were learning to operate unfamiliar equipment. The lesson to be learned was: When getting acquainted with a new instrument it is important to understand its "knobology"—What does each knob and button do and how do they interact with each other?

What my professor did was to have each student put an image on an oscilloscope. He then made us leave the room. He proceeded to turn knobs and push buttons until each image was buried somewhere inside the instrument. Our challenge for the day was to find the image!

His goal was to make sure that each student knew how every control on the instrument worked, and he achieved that goal. I have tried the same experiment with technicians during in-service training sessions and it has proven to be a very useful technique.

CONCLUDING REMARKS

Understanding the characteristics of the various ultrasound devices enables you to quickly learn to utilize any system you encounter. In addition, a further understanding of what can go wrong and which simple steps to take can go a long way in reducing unnecessary frustration and service calls.

CHAPTER 4

Axial Eye Length Measurements

Performing Axial Length Measurements

When performing an axial eye length measurement, there are a number of things to keep in mind. To be considered are the individual echoes and echo patterns along with the actual clinical techniques. In this chapter, the important aspects of what to look for and expect in an axial echogram as well as the various methods for obtaining measurements will be covered in detail.

There are three techniques used to perform axial eye length measurements. This chapter will discuss each method along with its advantages and disadvantages so that the most appropriate technique may be used. It is important to know all three methods because each has special applications. Most likely, one technique will be used for the majority of scans while one or both of the others would be utilized in special situations.

The axial length measurement is one of three key values used to calculate the power of a permanently implanted intraocular lens. Therefore, great care and consideration must be taken to ensure accurate results.

The three techniques are referred to as:

1. Immersion
2. Slit lamp applanation
3. Hand held applanation

These will be discussed in the order of desirability. It is true, however, that the vast majority of technicians and physicians utilize the second technique, slit lamp applanation. The first technique, immersion, is sometimes referred to as the purist method. It is my hope that the explanation of the immersion technique will inspire some of you to try this method and possibly incorporate it into your echographic examinations. Before delving into the various techniques for performing an axial length A-scan, I will offer a brief review of some of the fundamental principles that should be keep in mind during every examination.

Basic Principles Revisited

Many people have the mistaken idea that performing an axial eye length A-scan is about as simple as taking a patient's temperature. You simply put a probe on an eye, a machine beeps and the measurement in the display may be trusted as correct. Unfortunately, this is not the case. In order to have consistently accurate results, we must have an understanding of the reasons why we do what we do and why we see what we see on the screen. No ultrasound machine is smarter than its human operator.

As pointed out in the principles chapter, an A-scan is an echogram that is evaluated for its varying echo amplitudes. It is one-dimensional and utilizes a stationary transducer, called a probe. The varying heights of the echoes tell the examiner many things about the tissues that produced them. We know that the structures to be measured in this type of scan are generally considered to be highly reflective. This means that the sound reflects off of them quite well.

A good reflector of sound energy will therefore produce a tall echo when the sound beam is directed perpendicularly toward it. A short echo is displayed when the sound beam is not at a 90 degree angle to a strongly reflecting surface. This principle makes it easier to interpret an axial eye length A-scan because when the echoes are not tall and steeply rising we should assume that it is because the sound beam is not aligned properly with the ocular structures.

Interfaces Produce Echoes

Think about the surface of a structure in the eye as being an interface between two different types of tissue. It is this interface which actually creates reflected echoes. An echo

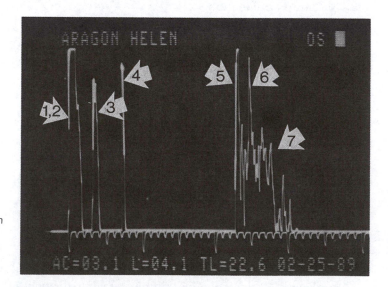

Figure 4.1 Classic pattern from an applanation axial length A-scan: cornea (1,2), anterior lens (3), posterior lens (4), retina (5), sclera (6), orbital fat (7).

from the lens in the eye is not produced because the lens is "hard" as some might think. In normal eyes and those with cataracts, the echoes that we wish to measure are produced by the interfaces between highly dissimilar tissues. This results in tall, strong reflections when the sound beam is aligned properly with these interfaces.

Ocular Echoes

There are many ocular echoes requiring our attention in an axial eye length A-scan. From anterior to posterior, they are:

PHAKIC EYE
1. Anterior cornea
2. Posterior cornea
3. Anterior lens capsule
4. Posterior lens capsule
5. Retina
6. Sclera
7. Orbital fat

APHAKIC EYE
1. Anterior cornea
2. Posterior cornea
3. Anterior vitreous face or posterior capsule (may or may not be present)
4. Retina
5. Sclera
6. Orbital fat

Cornea

The cornea produces the first echo of importance in an axial length A-scan. As you will see in the following sections, the displayed images of the cornea differ, depending upon the technique used. The corneal echo is the critically important point at which the measurement begins. Therefore, when checking the integrity of the corneal echo on any axial length scan, you must also verify that the instrument's measuring gate or caliper is properly positioned on the anterior surface of the echo. Later sections will discuss gates and their proper placement.

Corneal echoes have a strikingly different appearance in the immersion versus the applanation technique. In the immersion method, the individual echoes from the front and back corneal surfaces are clear. In the applanation method, the echo from the tip of the probe merges with echoes from the cornea to become a single broad echo.

The corneal echo is the only one to have a different appearance in the immersion technique than in the applanation technique. In the applanation technique, when the probe touches the cornea the echo from the tip of the probe and the echoes from the front and back of the cornea merge and become one and the same. This often presents a fairly thick echo when compared with other A-scan echoes.

In the immersion technique, separate echoes from both the anterior and posterior surfaces of the cornea will be visible. This corneal echo resembles the split end of a hair. In fact, it can be split all the way down to the base line of the scan. This echo will not, however, be the first one on

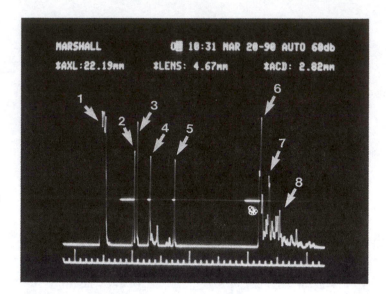

Figure 4.2 Classic pattern from an immersion axial length A-scan: probe tip (1), anterior cornea (2), posterior cornea (3), anterior lens (4), posterior lens (5), retina (6), sclera (7), orbital fat (8).

the screen, but will be the second echo. The first echo will come from the probe tip.

The double-peaked corneal echo is created because the resolution of the image is greater when the echo from the tip of the probe does not interfere with the echoes from the cornea. This can only be achieved by putting some distance between the probe and the cornea. This is accomplished by filling that space with a fluid that will transmit the sound. Therefore, the two interfaces in the cornea as seen in the immersion technique are between the fluid and the anterior surface, and the posterior surface and the aqueous.

Lens

Lens echoes can vary greatly from one patient to the next. Cataractous changes in the crystalline lens can cause extra reflections of sound. These extra echoes appear between the two "normal" echoes from the anterior and posterior lens surfaces.

The echo pattern from the lens as well as the remainder of the ocular echoes listed above is identical in both the immersion and applanation techniques. The normal, clear lens is homogeneous. This means that there are no significant interfaces between its front and back surfaces. The nucleus and the surrounding cortex of the lens are all similar tissues. On A-scans, this will produce one tall, strong echo from the interface between the aqueous and the anterior lens capsule, and one tall echo from the interface between the posterior lens capsule and the vitreous.

When looking at a drawing of the eye, it can be seen that both surfaces of the lens are curved, the posterior surface having a slightly greater curvature than the anterior sur-

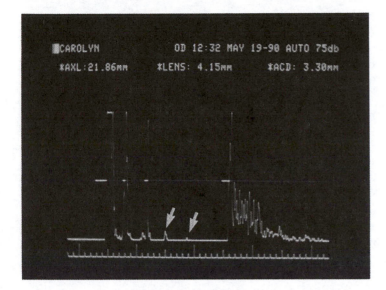

Figure 4.3 Two small reverberation echoes (arrows) from the clear crystalline lens. Note similar spacing to that of the lens echoes and that the second reverb is shorter than the first.

face. What this means to the examiner is that there is one orientation of the sound beam through the lens which is most desirable. This orientation is through the thickest portion, being perpendicular to both surfaces.

A small echo is sometimes displayed just past the posterior lens echo. This gives the appearance of there being something in the vitreous. Actually, it is an image of a type of artifact, or unwanted echo produced by reverberations of sound within the lens. This artifact can be useful, how-

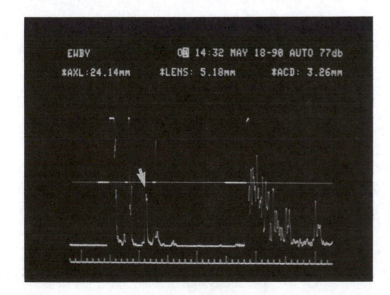

Figure 4.4 Arrow indicates an extra echo from within the lens produced by a cataract. Also note the small unevenly spaced echoes in the vitreous from floaters.

ever. When you see this in your scan, it can be used as a gauge of your sound beam alignment. The taller it is from one scan to the next for the same eye, the more perpendicular your sound beam is to both the anterior and posterior lens surfaces.

What happens when a cataract is present? A variety of things might occur, beginning with no apparent change in the echogram or a startling number of excess echoes in the scan. Think about the basic principles again. If the cataract development is causing changes within the lens material itself, it is logical to assume that some of these changes may produce interfaces of dissimilar tissues.

If the gain is turned too high, inaccurate readings can result. There are two ways to obtain a tall A-scan echo: one is to turn up the gain; the other is to align the probe correctly. High gain creates noise throughout the image which can mask a real ocular condition.

A common occurrence is that as a nuclear sclerotic cataract develops, the center, or nucleus, of the lens becomes opaque. Along with this opacification comes structural changes in the lens tissue. The ultrasound beam is sensitive and can often detect these changes. What will be seen on the screen are extra echoes in between the primary ones produced by the anterior and posterior lens surfaces.

Generally, the internal lens echoes are smaller than the primary ones. The echogram of just the nuclear sclerotic lens could present four echoes: (1) anterior lens capsule, (2) anterior nucleus, (3) posterior nucleus, and (4) posterior capsule. Therefore, do not be alarmed if a variety of extra echoes are produced from within the lens.

There is a point at which the extra echoes from the cataractous changes can cause problems for the examiner. This occurs when they interfere with the instrument's ability to measure the proper echoes. If the ultrasound unit has separate measuring gates for the lens, it will be important to see that these gates are in fact on the correct echoes, ensuring an accurate measurement. This is discussed in further detail later in this chapter in the section concerning what to look for in a phakic scan.

Vitreous

By now you should be able to explain why we see no echoes from normal vitreous. It is because there are no interfaces in the vitreous gel to produce a reflection. But what should you do if you see echoes from the vitreous? The physician should be notified of this or any other abnormal finding.

Small echoes from the vitreous could be produced by something as benign as floaters (slight opacifications or changes in the structure of the vitreous) or from something more serious like a vitreous hemorrhage. A fresh hemorrhage would result in very low echoes, possibly diffusely spread out along the base line. Why does blood in the vitreous produce short echoes? The reason is again explained through the application of basic principles.

The difference between fluid blood and the vitreous gel is very slight. It can be said that there is a small acoustic impedance at these interfaces. This small amount of dissimilarity produces small echoes. If blood has been in the eye for a longer period of time, it tends to become organized and, therefore, the interfaces become more significant, producing slightly taller echoes.

Ocular Disorders

I am often asked, "Will I see a retinal detachment or tumor on an axial length A-scan?" The answer is almost always no. A significant ocular disorder could possibly be present, but not show up on your A-scan. This is because the sound beam being sent into the eye for an axial length is directed through only one very small part of the globe. An extensive retinal detachment or other serious pathology could be present in a peripheral part of the globe, out of view of the A-scan sound beam. This is one reason for performing a diagnostic B-scan in cases where the physician cannot see through the cataract in order to evaluate the posterior and peripheral portions of the eye.

Retina

If forced to rate the importance of any individual echo in the axial length pattern, the retinal echo would have to be chosen as number one. Since the focal point of the eye lies at the macula, it is most critical to obtain a perfect echo from this region. What constitutes a perfect echo? The desirable quality is a tall, sharply rising echo.

Sharply rising means two things. First, there must be a 90 degree angle between the base line and the leading edge of the echo. The second essential aspect is that the left edge of the echo should be smooth and contain no ragged edges or stair steps. Anything other than a sharply rising, tall retinal echo indicates one of two things:

1. The sound beam is not perpendicular to the retina.
2. There may be pathology, such as a posterior vitreous membrane, hemorrhage, staphyloma, or other con-

Good perpendicularity between the sound beam and tissue is indicated by a sharply rising echo with a smooth left-hand edge. In an analog system, a sharply rising echo has a dim edge because it shoots up to the top of the screen so fast. In a digital system, the left edge may have a stair step profile.

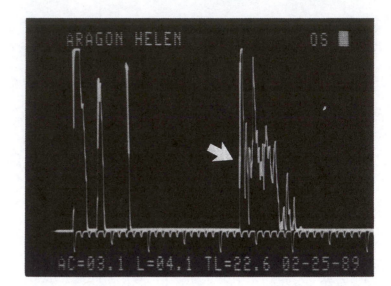

Figure 4.5 A good retinal echo, tall and sharply rising leading edge.

dition where the interface between the vitreous and retinal surface is not as significant as usual.

Staphyloma is a frequent cause of a poor retinal echo. A patient who has a high degree of myopia may exhibit a staphyloma, an abnormal shape to the globe. This means that the curvature of the retinal surface is not uniform and is often much more sharply curved than a normal eye. The difference in curvature may be illustrated this way: The normal eye's posterior shape is like the large end of an egg,

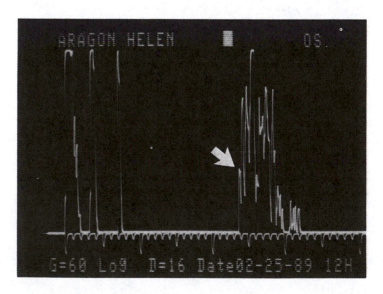

Figure 4.6 A poor retinal echo, not tall and steeply rising.

whereas the eye with a staphyloma is often like the more pointed end of the egg.

Some staphylomas, however, may have multiple curvatures in the posterior segment of the eye making it nearly impossible to obtain a valid axial length scan. In these eyes, it is difficult to determine where the macula is located. As will be covered in more detail later, determining the measurement to the macula is our highest goal.

Sclera and Orbital Fat

The actual measurement of axial length is the distance from the cornea to the retina along the visual axis. So why worry about echoes from the sclera and orbital fat? There are specific reasons why additional echoes from the tissues posterior to the retina must be visible in the scan before it is to be considered valid.

There should always be an echo complex (several echoes in a group) from the back of the eye. These include the retinal, scleral, and orbital fat signals. It is never sufficient to have only one echo from the posterior segment. The thought behind this statement is that if there is only one echo, how do you know that it is really the retina? If there are echoes from the retina, sclera, and orbital fat, then the first one of the group should be the retina.

In addition to using the other posterior echoes as indicators that the one being measured is the retina, there is a clinical significance as well. The sound beam directed toward the macula is the correct axial length of the eye. Think about what is directly behind the macula. The sclera and orbital fat are posterior to the retina in the macular region. The choroid is not very reflective of ultrasound when it is in its normal position between the retina and sclera. Therefore, we do not clearly see a separate choroidal echo.

The sclera is actually the most reflective tissue in the eye, so we should expect to see a strong echo from it. Directly behind the sclera in the macular region, there is orbital fat. Therefore, a complete axial eye length scan will include a complex of echoes from the posterior pole including retina, sclera, and orbital fat.

Two factors could result in an echogram having only one echo from the posterior pole. First, it could be that the sound beam is not perpendicular to the retinal surface but is perpendicular to the highly reflective sclera. A measurement from this kind of scan would be too long and of course inaccurate, since the sclera is behind the retina.

It is not good enough to have just one tall echo from the back of the eye. The retinal echo must be followed by those from the sclera and orbital fat. We know that there are tissues behind the macula, so corresponding echoes should be displayed.

There is a second and very common cause of only one echo being produced from the posterior segment. The sound beam could be directed toward the optic disk, where the optic nerve exits the eye. When you think about it, there are no scleral or orbital fat echoes right behind the disk, since the optic nerve is there. Consequently, even though the scleral and orbital fat echoes are not used for measuring, they are still very important to ensure the validity of the scan.

Measuring Gates

The purpose of a measuring gate or caliper or overlight is to indicate to the examiner which echoes on the screen are being measured by the instrument. Each manufacturer has its own way of doing things and it will be necessary to study the specifics of your instrument's gates in the instruction manual that came with the unit.

Some gates are movable and others are fixed. Still others are visible, while others are invisible. My preference is to have visible and movable gates so that the operator has the maximum control over the image. There are various ways in which the gates may appear on the screen:

1. A horizontal line positioned under the echoes to be measured
2. A horizontal line touching the leading edge of the echo

Practice moving the measuring cursors or gates. Notice that small or large movements create significant changes in the reading. The knowledge of how to quickly and accurately move the gates may prove important while scanning difficult cases.

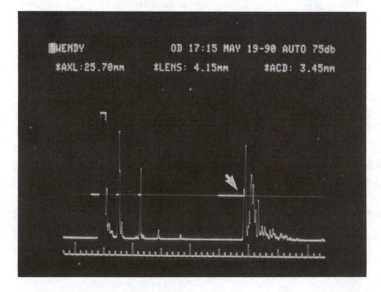

Figure 4.7 Correct retinal gate placement is on first part of echo's leading or rising edge. Note measurement of 25.70 mm.

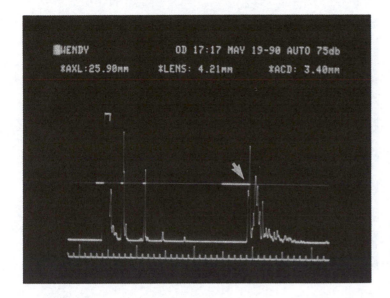

Figure 4.8 Incorrect retinal gate placement on the higher part of the echo past steeply rising edge shows an increase in measurement of 0.20 mm.

3. A vertical line to the left of the echo
4. A bright dot or line that traces the outline of the echo

You should practice maneuvering the gates on your instrument so that when it is necessary to move one in the middle of a scan, it may be done quickly.

The number of gates available on a unit is often dependent upon the type of eye being measured. For example, one type of instrument has four gates for phakic scans, three for pseudophakic, and two for aphakic and miscellaneous structure measurements.

What to Look for in a Phakic Scan

In an eye that is phakic (one with a natural lens), the requirements of a good scan are:

1. Tall echo from the cornea, one echo in the contact technique and a double-peaked echo in the immersion technique
2. Tall echoes from the anterior and posterior lens
3. Tall, sharply rising echo from the retina
4. Medium tall to tall echo from the sclera
5. Medium to low echoes from the orbital fat

In contrast, an unacceptable A-scan may include:

1. One or more echoes of insufficient amplitude
2. Retinal echo rising up from the base line at a slope

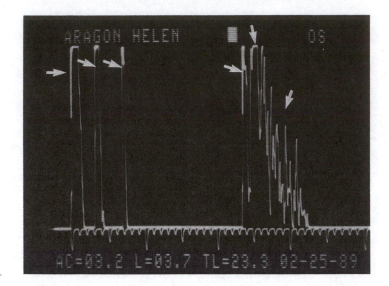

Figure 4.9 A classic phakic scan, all echoes are clearly defined, tall, and steeply rising.

3. Retinal echo fairly steep, but with a jagged edge
4. Only one echo from the back of the eye

One or more of these conditions could result in rejecting the scan, but a touch of reality is appropriate here. There will be challenging cases out there just waiting to test your patience. Sometimes there is no maneuvering of the probe that will produce a classic scan. Therefore, a compromise must be made.

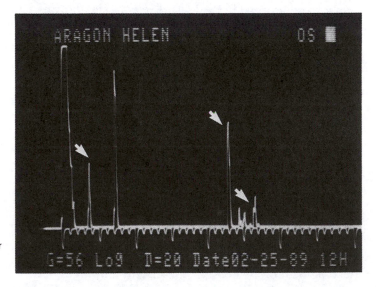

Figure 4.10 A poor phakic scan shows insufficient anterior lens, retinal, scleral, and orbital fat echoes.

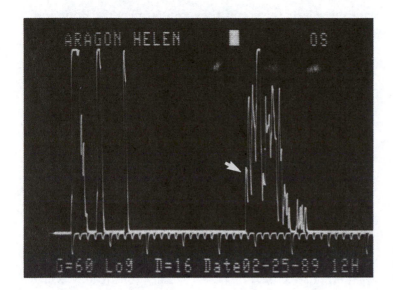

Figure 4.11 A poor phakic scan has ragged edge of retinal echo, not steeply rising.

In order of priority, judge a scan first by the qualities of a sharply rising retinal echo with a scleral echo as well. If the posterior echoes are great but the lens echoes aren't both tall, the scan is most likely adequate.

A scan with two tall lens echoes and a medium height retinal echo would be adequate and not acceptable. Try again, and concentrate on the retinal and scleral signals.

Another difficulty can occur with the placement of lens gates. If the gate for the posterior capsule echo is attached to one of the internal echoes of the lens, the displayed lens thickness will be falsely short. When an instrument measures the lens incorrectly, it can cause an error in the overall length due to the difference in sound velocities between the different tissues. If possible, correct the situation by moving the posterior lens gate to the actual posterior lens echo.

If the gates are neither visible nor movable, try repeating the scan with slightly lower gain. The lower gain may reduce any interference caused by internal cataract echoes.

Producing echoes of relatively equal amplitude is more important than having all of them reach the top of the screen.

As with any type of axial length scan, being able to reproduce both the scan quality as well as the measurement is a requirement. I have often been shown several scans that vary in echo pattern quality and measurement. The question is asked, "Which one should I choose?" The answer is usually, "None of them." If you cannot reproduce the scan and the measurement, it is not valid.

It doesn't matter how many scans the instrument automatically selects for you if they do not meet the minimum requirements with respect to echo quality and measurement reproducibility. Keep scanning until you are confident with all of the results.

Be certain that the instrument is programmed for phakic. This will mean dialing in an average phakic velocity of 1548 or 1550 m/s, as with some older units, or selecting phakic from a menu in most of the newer models.

When phakic is selected as a menu choice, there are two velocity methods an instrument may utilize when making a measurement:

1. A calculated ratio of the aqueous/vitreous and lens velocities which produces an average of 1548 or 1550 m/s
2. Individual measurements of each ocular structure, 1532 m/s for aqueous/vitreous and 1641 m/s for lens (although some units use 1620 m/s for the lens, which produces an insignificant difference)

What to Look for in an Aphakic Scan

In the case of an aphakic patient (one having no natural lens), directing the sound beam toward the macula is even more critical, as there are no lens echoes to help indicate sound beam alignment along the axis.

Occasionally there will be an echo in the location where

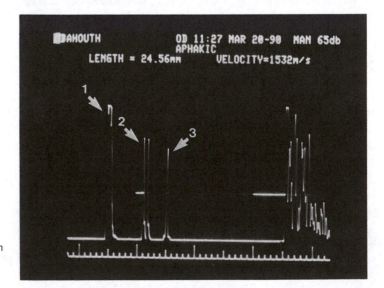

Figure 4.12 A classic immersion aphakic scan. Echoes displayed are from probe tip (1), double echo of anterior and posterior cornea (2), and posterior capsule left in the eye after the cataract was removed (3).

the posterior lens capsule would normally be. This can be one of two things. It could be an echo from the posterior capsule which has been left intact after the removal of the lens. The extra echo could also arise from the interface between the aqueous and vitreous.

There is only a small difference in acoustic impedance between the aqueous and vitreous. This makes sense, since these ocular fluids are so similar. If there is an echo produced by this interface, it will most likely be small and much less stable than echoes from other structures. It may be visible one instant and invisible the next.

Remember to make certain that the correct velocity of 1532 m/s is being used to calculate the axial length. Since there is no lens in the aphakic eye, it is imperative that the sound velocity be verified. In some instruments, this is done by dialing in the speed on the front panel. Other units have a switch to flip down for aphakic measurements, while still others make the eye type selection with the computer keyboard or with a light pen. Since the majority of eyes being measured for IOL calculations are phakic, be extra careful to return the instrument to the proper phakic settings prior to evaluating the next patient.

Sometimes aphakic eyes produce an echo where the lens used to be. This can be caused by the posterior capsule in the case of an extracapsular cataract extraction, or the interface between aqueous and vitreous in the event of an intracapsular extraction.

What to Look for in a Pseudophakic Scan

Pseudophakic eyes present very different echoes. In eyes with an IOL already in place, there will be additional echoes created by the sound beam reverberating between the plastic lens and the probe. The primary reason for this is that the interface between the aqueous and the anterior surface of the implant is very significant, thereby producing a strong reflection of sound energy. In fact, it is usually necessary to turn down the gain. This will help reduce the reverberation echoes so that the retinal and scleral echoes may be clearly seen.

Great care must be taken when measuring a postoperative eye. First, find out when the surgery was performed. Needless to say, a contact A-scan is not advisable in the early post-op period. Consult with the physician prior to the scan if in doubt. Next, see that the gain is high enough to obtain a retinal echo, yet low enough to reduce reverberations. There can be so many echoes in the eye that determining which one is the retina can be a challenge.

Lastly, determine of what material the IOL was made. The reason for this is again a velocity issue to be discussed next.

Watch out for a multitude of extra echoes when scanning a pseudophakic eye with an IOL. These reverberation echoes can interfere with measuring the retina. Turn down the gain to sort through the echoes.

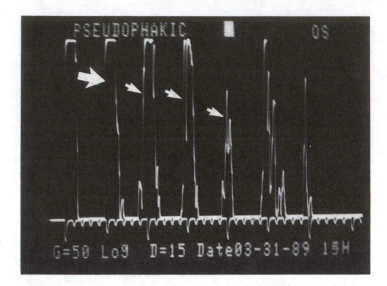

Figure 4.13 A classic pseudophakic (PMMA) axial length scan. The large arrow indicates the IOL echo; smaller three arrows show reverberations.

Pseudophakic PMMA IOLs

The velocity of sound must definitely be taken into consideration when measuring the pseudophakic eye. Until just recently, the vast majority of IOLs have been made from polymethylmethacrylate (PMMA). This type of plastic has a very high sound velocity and consequently there are well-established methods for measuring such eyes.

An older method is to measure the eye with the average velocity of 1550 m/s to obtain a reasonably accurate result. Another

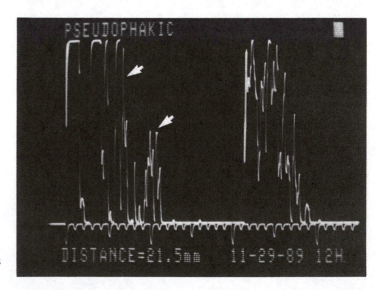

Figure 4.14 Another pseudophakic scan with arrows indicating reverbs from IOL.

common method is to measure the eye as if it were aphakic, by using 1532 m/s and then adding a compensating value to that result. The most frequently used compensating value is 0.23 mm.

For example, if the pseudophakic eye measures 23.75 mm using the aphakic velocity, add 0.23 mm to that result to obtain a corrected axial length of 23.98 mm. It is impossible, however, to be a hundred percent accurate in this type of postoperative measurement because we cannot truly measure the IOL thickness. The IOL thickness changes slightly with the different implant lens powers, and this can have an effect on the measured axial length.

Most of the newer instruments have built-in programs for measuring the length of an eye with an IOL in place. They generally use one of the methods mentioned above. Consult the instruction manual or check with the company for details.

Pseudophakic Silicone IOLs

There is a new player in the IOL field—an IOL made of silicone. It is generally used so that it may be folded to fit through a smaller incision site. The presence of this type of IOL in the eye will produce a dramatic difference in the post-op measurement as compared to the pre-op readings.

If the instrument you use has a program for pseudophakic measurements, unless it says otherwise you can safely assume that it is set up for measuring eyes with implants made from PMMA. The silicone IOLs are still under study, but will undoubtedly be readily available in the near future. Therefore, we must be prepared to deal with this situation.

The determination of the proper velocity to use for this type of postoperative measurement has been documented by Albert T. Milauskas, MD, and Sherrie Marney, CRA. (See *Journal of Cataract and Refractive Surgery*, Volume 14, Number 4, pages 400–402.) What they found was an apparent increase in the postoperative axial length of eyes implanted with a lens made of RMX-3 silicone. This increase was approximately 1 mm.

This significant deviation from the preoperative measurements prompted them to conduct a study. An immersion A-scan measurement of a one-centimeter-thick test block of silicone was made using the aphakic mode in their instrument. This mode presented two measuring gates on the screen. One was positioned on the echo from the top surface of the silicone and the second gate on the echo from

The new silicone IOLs cause a postoperative axial length that is longer by about 1 mm than the preoperative measurement. This is due to the fact that ultrasound travels very slowly through silicone. Either modify the measurement later, or if your unit is programmable, be certain that the correct velocities have been selected.

the bottom of the block. That measurement was placed into an algebraic formula and the velocity of 1049 m/s for the silicone was obtained. They also determined that an average velocity of 1486 m/s may be used to obtain the correct postoperative axial length.

If the ultrasound instrument cannot be reprogrammed with this new velocity, the following procedure should be followed:

1. Measure the eye with the aphakic velocity of 1532 m/s.
2. Multiply the falsely long measurement by a correcting factor of 0.96 to obtain the correct value.

For example, if an eye with a silicone lens measures 23.50 mm, that value multiplied by a factor of 0.96 will result in a corrected axial length of 22.56 mm. As you can see, this makes a considerable difference. As will be discussed further in the chapter covering ocular relationships:

1 millimeter in axial length = 3 diopters in refraction

This is a potentially dangerous problem due to the fact that a patient may have an unknown IOL in place. Patients rarely know the details of their surgery and their records may not be available. In a case encountered by Dr. Milauskas, he was presented with the challenge of having to remove a decentered silicone lens and replace it with a PMMA lens. In order to calculate the correct power for the new PMMA implant, a valid axial length was required. Had the doctor not known the original preoperative length and had the technician not noticed the discrepancy not only between the pre- and postoperative measurements, but also between the measurements of both eyes, the patient could have ended up with a three diopter error in postoperative refraction.

If Milauskas and Marney's original article is reviewed, please note that there is a typographical error on page 401. The aphakic velocity in the instrument they used was 1532 m/s, not 1550 as written.

As you can see, new developments in IOL material and design will affect those of us who are taking the responsibility for accurately measuring these eyes. Now we must ask a new question when scanning a pseudophakic patient, "Of what material is the implant made?"

Techniques Common to All Methods

Before delving into the various techniques for performing an axial length A-scan, it will be helpful to briefly review some of the concepts that are the same for all methods.

Topical Anesthetic

A topical anesthetic is of course needed for every technique of axial length measurement to numb the cornea for a few minutes while the test is being performed. Follow the manufacturer's instructions and warnings and do not use the solution if it becomes discolored or if the dropper tip of the bottle becomes contaminated. Check the expiration date also. When instilling drops, have the patient look up and allow the drop to go into the lower lid. This is more comfortable for the patient, and making them happy right from the start can only help.

Making the Patient Comfortable

It does not seem that this subject would need to be addressed, but I have observed numerous situations in which the patient's comfort was not properly considered. The fundamental idea is that if the patient is physically comfortable, they will be more likely to cooperate with the examiner. It is true that some patients are complainers, no matter how much we might try to accommodate them, but generally speaking, patients need to be asked if they are comfortable. They are often reluctant to admit that they are miserable.

Keeping the patient physically as well as emotionally comfortable will greatly enhance your ability to perform a biometric measurement. Unhappy patients are not known for being cooperative.

A patient's aching neck or back, or a poorly adjusted slit lamp can make the difference between a quick, complete exam, or a tedious and incomplete one. Have you ever noticed how cold the forehead and chin rests can get on one of those A-scan applanation stands? I have always been a proponent of having technicians perform these exams on each other so that they may be more sensitive to the patient's needs. When in doubt, ask the patient if they are comfortable and instruct them to tell you if they are not.

Cleaning the Probes

Any solid-tipped A-scan probe may be cleaned with an alcohol prep pad, or soaked in the Clinic Alert solution in the manner recommended by the Center for Disease Control.

The purpose of using this solution is to dramatically reduce or eliminate HIV infectious agents. The HIV virus is carried by AIDS patients. An article in *Argus*, November 1988, page 25, thoroughly explains the role of HIV infection precautions in the ophthalmic setting. The title of the article is "Updated Recommendations for Ophthalmic Practice in Relation to the Human Immunodeficiency Virus." I rec-

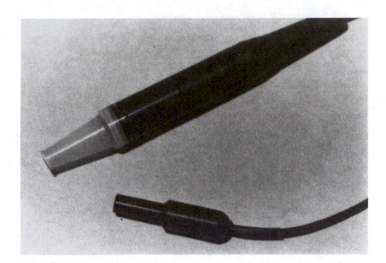

Figure 4.15 Two examples of biometry probes; longer fluid-filled probe fits in chin rest, smaller solid one fits in a tonometer.

ommend that all ophthalmic personnel obtain a copy of this important article and keep it for reference. Copies are available from the American Academy of Ophthalmology in San Francisco, (415) 561-8500.

Basically, this article states that given the low risk of transmitting HIV through contact with tears, the proven efficacy of simply cleaning tonometer tips well with an alcohol sponge will eliminate the herpes virus and may provide adequate protection against HIV as well.

If you are not sure that the probe was properly cleaned after the last patient was examined, take the time to do it before the next exam. Solid probes may be cleaned with an alcohol prep, then rinsed with sterile saline.

If alcohol is used, it is recommended that the tip of the instrument be cleaned immediately after each patient and allowed to dry for at least 1 to 2 minutes before the next

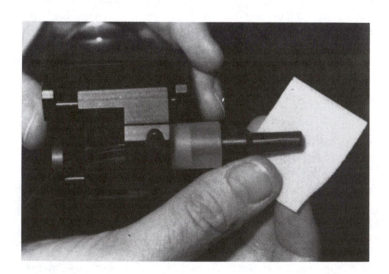

Figure 4.16 Clean tip with alcohol swab between patients.

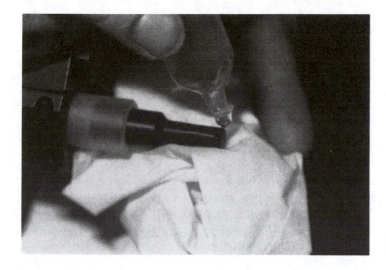

Figure 4.17 *Rinse residual alcohol with sterile saline.*

scan. Some institutions require that sterile saline be used after the alcohol to ensure that no residue remains.

The Clinic Alert method calls for soaking the first 2 to 3 mm of the instrument's tip for a period of 5 to 10 minutes. The two approved solutions are:

1. Full-strength 3% hydrogen peroxide
2. A 1:10 dilution of household bleach

After the soaking, the probes are to be rinsed with tap water or sterile saline and dried.

When preparing the first solution listed above, use full-strength 3% hydrogen peroxide. The peroxide solution must be changed two times each day. Obviously, the probe should be unplugged from the console and the connector must never come in contact with water.

The second solution is a 1:10 dilution of household bleach. For a 1:10 dilution, one part bleach is mixed with 10 parts distilled water. The bleach solution must be replaced once each day.

In the *Archives of Ophthalmology*, Volume 106, November 1988, page 1505, there is a case report demonstrating a corneal toxicity from a hydrogen peroxide-soaked tonometer tip which apparently was in a solution that had evaporated. This evaporation apparently caused a change in the concentration of the solution, producing a reaction with the tip of the tonometer. A properly soaked and rinsed probe tip should not cause a problem with the cornea.

The cleaning of membrane-tipped, water-filled A-scan probes presents a major difficulty since there is no way to effectively clean the membranes. There is a risk that the cleaning agents will be absorbed into the pores of the membrane and then be transferred onto the cornea. When in doubt about the cleanliness of the membrane, just replace it. At a minimum, irrigate the tip with sterile saline after each patient and again prior to the next.

Reducing Distractions

It is difficult enough for a calm person to hold their eyes in a fixed gaze without having to cope with distractions. But during ultrasound examinations, we require a great deal of cooperation from patients who may be nervous or frightened. Reducing distractions can make a big difference in how well they cooperate.

Begin by dimming the room lights. This will allow the patient to fixate on a target, either the light inside the probe or another type of target. Try to position the patient so that they are not facing an open doorway. People walking by can cause the patient to look up, no matter how hard they are trying to concentrate for you. If possible, close the door. By providing a calm, quiet atmosphere, both you and the patient will complete the tasks at hand more quickly and efficiently.

IMMERSION

In the immersion technique, the probe never touches the cornea. Consequently, there is no worry about corneal compression. After taking a little time to become acquainted with the technique, many feel it can be performed just as quickly as the applanation method since reproducibility of the measurements is usually greater.

The unique feature about the immersion method is that the ultrasound probe never actually touches the eye. This has value since one of the most common errors made while performing an applanation (contact) axial eye length A-scan is the compression or flattening of the cornea, producing a falsely short measurement. In fact, the word applanation itself has to do with the concept of flattening.

The three fundamental advantages of the immersion method are:

1. Not touching the cornea prevents inaccuracies due to corneal compression.
2. Reproducibility of the measurement is more readily obtained.
3. Echoes from the cornea are useful in aligning the sound beam along the visual axis, providing additional assurance of a measurement to the macula.

Special Equipment

Performing this examination requires some special equipment such as a scleral shell, possibly a different probe, certain solutions, a particular type of reclining exam chair, and a fellow eye fixation target.

Scleral Shells

A special eye cup, commonly called a scleral shell, is required for performing the immersion technique axial eye length scan. The shells are cylinders of plastic with one edge flared out slightly, similar to the bell of a trumpet. This allows it to fit comfortably on the anesthetized sclera under the patient's lids.

One common type comes in a set containing shells of several different diameters. This allows the examiner to choose an appropriate size to fit a range of palpebral fissures (eyelid openings). There are two different sets of shells. One is a set of three, containing shells with 20, 22, and 24 mm diameters. The other set has these same three plus two smaller ones, 16 and 18 mm. The set of three is adequate for adult eyes.

These scleral shell sets are available only from Hansen Ophthalmic Development Labs, P.O. Box 613, Iowa City, IA 52244, (319) 338-1285. The prices vary depending upon which set is ordered. Single replacement shells may be purchased separately.

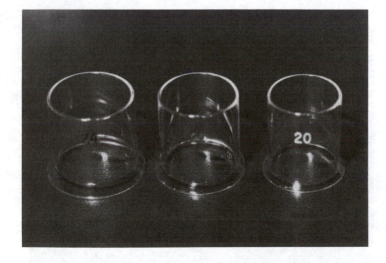

Figure 4.18 Immersion shells, set of three different sizes.

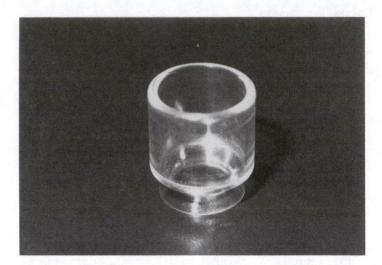

Figure 4.19 Immersion shell, one size fits all.

Other shells have a custom design for a specific type of probe. One of these shown was designed by Thomas Prager, PhD, of the University of Texas, Houston. It is made specifically for the Biophysic/Alcon axial length probe and is available through Alcon. It may be available for other A-scan probes in the future.

Dr. Prager designed these shells in order to increase the accuracy and reproducibility of axial length measurements obtained from a number of different technicians in their clinic. In this shell, the probe is secured with small set screws and saline is injected through the filling shaft located on the side of the shell. There are holes inside for the air to escape while the saline is being injected.

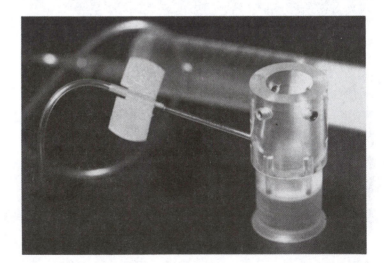

Figure 4.20 Immersion shell, custom made for a specific probe with side port to inject fluid.

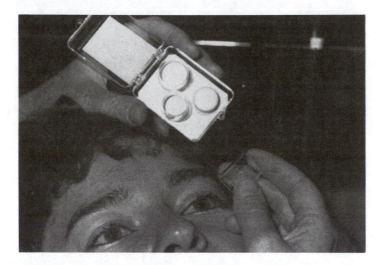

Figure 4.21. Selecting the appropriate diameter shell based on the patient's fissure.

Yet another shell is a "one size fits all" type, having a base with a very broad flange. It will accommodate various sizes of eye fissures. This is available from Eye Associates of Sebastopol Medical Group, Inc., attention Laura Darling, P.O. Box 1777, Sebastopol, CA 94573.

Care of Scleral Shells

When the shell is removed from the eye (details in technique will be covered next), it is usually placed on a tissue. Care should be taken, however, that it is not accidentally thrown away with the tissue. One method of helping to

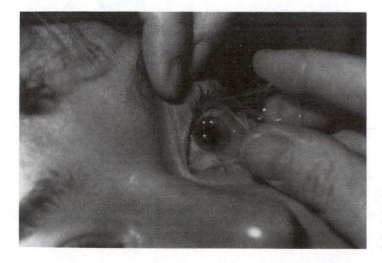

Figure 4.22 Lift the lid to position the flared edge of the shell on the sclera; instruct the patient to keep both eyes open.

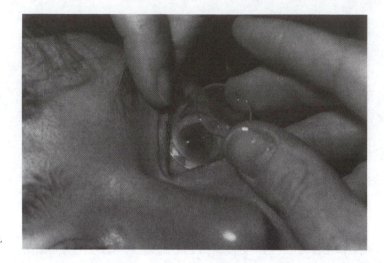

Figure 4.23 Shell is properly positioned on anesthetized eye, cornea in center.

avoid this is to paint a band around the outer part of the shell with brightly colored nail polish. This will survive the constant cleaning and disinfecting of the shells. Most people simply wash and dry the shell after each examination, using mild soap and water. The shell may also be wiped with an alcohol prep pad or disinfected by being placed in the Clinic Alert solution for the required time and then rinsed.

Probe and Fixation Light

Some physicians feel that with the immersion technique, a special probe should be used as well. This would be a par-

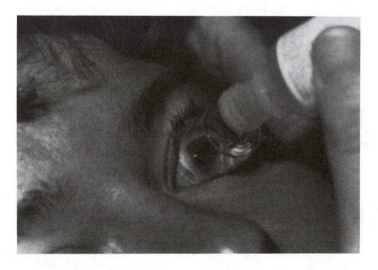

Figure 4.24 Pour sterile 2.5% methylcellulose onto inside surface of shell to help avoid bubbles. Note that dropper tip has been removed.

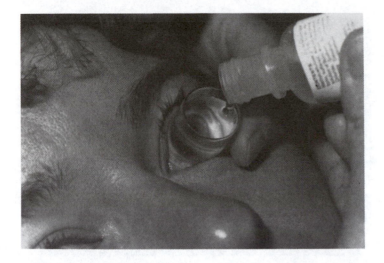

Figure 4.25 Fill shell almost to top of shell to allow for changes in probe depth.

allel beam probe, such as the one used for performing a standardized diagnostic A-scan. Others feel that the normal focused A-scan probe that is commonly used in the applanation method provides adequate results when used in the immersion technique.

The presence of an internal fixation light is not an important issue with this method since the fluid used in the shell prevents the patient from being able to see the light clearly. If saline is used instead of gel, then perhaps a fixation light built into the probe would be of use. In either case, it is more useful to have some sort of target for the patient to look at with the fellow eye. Examples of these are either a large X on the ceiling, since the patient is reclined, or better

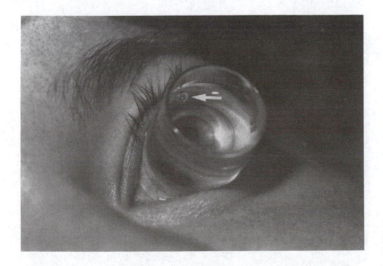

Figure 4.26 Small bubble off to the side and not in the path of the sound beam is tolerated.

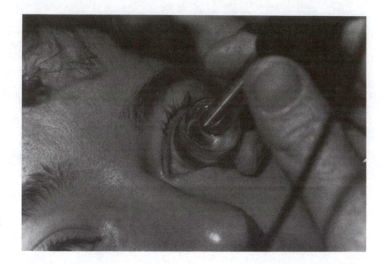

Figure 4.27 *Immersion probe is held near tip and hand is resting on cheek for stability. Sound beam is directed through center of pupil and toward macula. Tip of probe is immersed in the gel a few millimeters.*

yet, a movable red light fixation target that is either mounted to the back of the exam chair or to the ceiling. Even a bright poster mounted on the ceiling serves well.

Solutions

Solutions to have on hand are:

1. Topical anesthetic
2. Sterile methylcellulose 2.5% solution, generally used for gonioscopic examinations
3. Sterile unpreserved balanced saline (do not use saline in aerosol cans)
4. Comfort drops of some sort

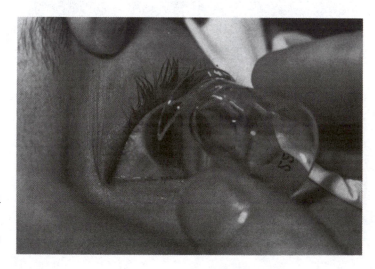

Figure 4.28 *Keep tissue near lateral canthus and lift up on lid when gently removing shell. Patient then closes the eye pushing out gel. Eye is then thoroughly irrigated with sterile saline.*

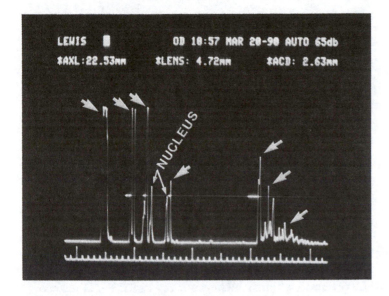

Figure 4.29 Immersion A-scan shows: probe tip, double peaked cornea, anterior lens, anterior nucleus, posterior nucleus, posterior lens, retina, sclera, and orbital fat.

Watch out for preservatives in the solutions that may cause an allergic reaction in the patient, and always check the expiration date on the containers.

When obtaining methylcellulose, carefully read the label and get the 2.5% concentration. The thicker consistency of the 2.5% solution makes it less likely to leak out of the shell. Sterile irrigating saline should be used to rinse the gel from the patient's eye after the measurement.

Remember that the patient's cornea ' ~en anesthetized during the immersion scan and h ᵇlinking function. Instruct the patient to keer ' for

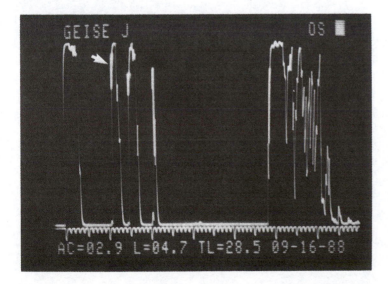

Figure 4.30 Another immersion A-scan showing probe tip separate from ocular echoes. The corneal echo is indicated by the arrow.

a few minutes after the exam. Warn the patient that the tear film balance has been disrupted by the examination procedure and that "the natural balance will re-establish itself shortly." Tell them you are instilling a drop of a tear substitute (Celluvisc works well) "to begin the process." Give the patient a sample of unpreserved artificial tears to use at home. As with all special tests, be solicitous of the patient's comfort.

Reclining Exam Chair

In order to position the patient comfortably as well as to provide the optimum setup for the examiner, a reclining examination chair is desirable. Personally, I prefer the type that keeps the patient seated while reclined. Patients in this type of chair do not complain about their back hurting as they often do when stretched out on a gurney. If a gurney or other flat examining table is all that is available, be sure to have a large pillow handy for placing under the patient's knees. There is nothing worse for a patient with a weak lower back than to have to lie perfectly flat.

Also, after the exam, when the patient sits up, allow them to stay seated for a couple of minutes, or until they feel ready to stand up. Sometimes a patient may feel dizzy when they first sit up. This is another reason for using a chair that tilts back while keeping the patient seated. When the chair is placed in the upright position again, the patient is more secure and not likely to fall while taking a minute or two to prepare themselves for getting out of the chair.

Preparing the Instrument

Some ultrasound units cannot be used for this technique, so check first with the manufacturer for details. The instrument will need to be adjusted differently for the immersion technique than for applanation. In units that have a computer-type menu, this may be a matter of simply selecting the examination method from a list. In the analog units (ones without a computer base or freeze frame capability), it usually means that the horizontal position of the image on the screen will need to be shifted so that all of the echoes will appear on the screen. The horizontal position of echoes is different for immersion than for applanation.

The echoes on the screen should not be so compressed that the entire A-scan takes up only one-half or one-third of the display, nor should they be so expanded that any echo is at the edge or off the edge of the screen. You will have to experiment with your instrument to see which position of the horizontal and magnification controls will allow the scan to be properly positioned. Check in the instrument's instruction manual for more specific details.

Be sure to note the correct sound velocities for each and every category of eye. Phakic, aphakic, and pseudophakic eyes have different speeds of sound which apply. These velocities have already been covered in earlier sections.

Lastly, position the screen of the instrument as close to the patient's head as possible. The examiner should only have to shift their gaze from the patient to the screen, not turn their head to look.

Preparing the Patient

The patient should be told in simple terms what to expect during this test. Here is an example: "I am going to take a measurement of your eye that will assist the doctor in selecting the correct intraocular lens for your cataract surgery. I will be measuring both of your eyes. Since your eyes work as a team, it is important for the doctor to look at the measurements from both eyes when preparing for your operation. In which eye are you having surgery?" It is always important to double- and triple- check this obviously important bit of information. If the patient is not consulted and you begin measuring the right eye first when it is the left one that is having surgery, they can get quite upset. If you look at the matter from their perspective, it appears as if they are about to get the wrong eye measured. In addition, talking to the patient makes them feel more like they are participating in this event.

To continue: "Let me explain what will happen in this test. I will have you lie back in this chair and look straight up at the ceiling. Next, I will put a drop in each eye that will make the surface of the eye numb for a few minutes. This will make you feel more comfortable. This drop does not dilate your pupils." It is amazing how many patients are worried about having their eyes dilated.

"Next I will be putting this little cup under your eyelids and will fill it with a cool liquid. I will ask you to keep both eyes open during the test. This little probe will send gentle sound waves into your eye, and the information I need will appear on this screen. You may hear the sound of the camera as I take some pictures. Be sure and let me know if you are uncomfortable, and I will do my best to help you. Do you have any questions?"

Be sure to talk to the patient— they're human and need attention. A little consideration can go a long way. Think of the patient as being your grandmother or uncle. Realize that they have their own worries that could be causing an inability to cooperate.

At this point, answer any questions they might have, and recline the chair. Be certain that the patient's head and neck are comfortable. They cannot help you by cooperating and following your instructions if they are miserable. Instill a topical anesthetic in each eye using the normal technique. Ask the patient to look up toward the top of their head, gently pull down on the lower lid and instill one drop into each eye. Wait a few seconds and instill a second drop in each eye. Insert the scleral shell by having them look down while the shell is slipped under the upper lid. Next, have the patient look straight up toward the ceiling and pull the lower lid away from and then over the edge of the shell. Press an absorbant towel against the patient's face by the temporal corner of the eye being examined. This will absorb any leakage of fluid and is a particularly important precaution if the patient is wearing a hearing aid.

This is now the time to remind them to keep both eyes open during the test. If they squeeze either their fellow eye or the eye being examined, it only accentuates the unusual feeling that they cannot close the eye in which the shell is placed; this may also cause the shell to pop out. It helps to touch your finger to the patient's temple next to the follow eye and say, "Keep this eye wide open and you will be more comfortable."

For filling the shell I prefer using methylcellulose gel, 2.5% concentration, as mentioned above in the section on solutions. It is nice and thick and won't leak out under the edges of the shell. Common brand names are Gonak and Goniosol. It is usually referred to as a gonioscopic solution. When using 2.5% methylcellulose, it is important to avoid getting air bubbles in the solution that could turn up in the gel once it is in the shell. The simplest way to do this is to remove the nipple from the bottle and just pour the solution out.

A 1% methylcellulose solution is also available, but I feel it is too thin. Some examiners use a combination of methylcellulose gel and sterile saline. They put a small amount of gel into the shell first, which acts as a seal around the edges, then they fill up the shell the rest of the way with sterile saline.

Even with the saline, however, it is important to be careful not to agitate the solution by squirting it in with too much force. Either take the nipple off the irrigating bottle and gently pour the solution, or direct the stream against the side of the shell and do not squeeze the bottle too hard. These techniques will avoid creating bubbles in the solution. Another type of saline in use is the kind that comes in individual nonreusable bottles. The reason I like this kind is that the solution does not come out of the bottle with so much force. The flow is more gentle since the opening at the tip is larger and a fresh, sterile bottle can be used for each patient.

There are still others who use only saline in the shell, and if it leaks, then they switch to gel. Personally, I have not had as much success using just saline since leakage is so often a problem. With the methylcellulose gel, I never have to worry because I know that it won't leak and that it will work well the first time. I would recommend trying the different techniques, however, to see what works best for you. Certainly there is a major advantage in using saline since it is significantly less expensive than methylcellulose and need not be rinsed out. The Prager shell is designed for using saline and leakage is generally not a problem.

In any case, fill the shell all the way to the top so that you have more flexibility in positioning the probe. It is important to be sure that the probe does not go so deep into the shell that it might come in contact with the cornea. It might seem at this point that the technician needs three hands to perform immersion A-scans. However, with a bit of practice it becomes easier to hold the towel and shell while balancing the probe. Don't give up, the results are worth the effort.

Evaluating Immersion Echoes

It is essential when evaluating the echo pattern on the screen to be able to clearly see the separation between the echo from the tip of the probe and the echoes from the cornea. The reason for being so concerned about this is that the axial length measurement is the distance from the anterior cornea to the anterior retina. It is the examiner's job to be certain that the first measuring gate or caliper is placed only on the anterior corneal echo. If the probe were too deep in the shell, the echo from the probe tip might be too close to the echoes from the cornea making it difficult to place the measuring gate correctly. Also, if the instrument is taking an automatic measurement, you want to be sure to note where the measurement begins.

When the probe is moved down toward the cornea, the entire echo pattern from the eye will shift toward the left of the screen. An undesirable effect of having the probe too deep in the shell is that the echoes could possibly shift so far that one or more of the anterior segment echoes (cornea, anterior lens or posterior lens) could be displaced off the screen. Sometimes a slight repositioning of the probe toward or away from the cornea is advantageous. This allows you to realign the image on the screen so that the echoes are in the proper position with respect to the measuring gates. This will depend somewhat on the specific ultrasound instrument being used.

If no measurement is displayed even when it appears that all of the echoes are correct, it may be that the gates are not in the correct position or that the scan pattern needs to be shifted slightly toward the gates. This happens more frequently in the immersion technique because of the ability of the operator to move the image by varying the depth of the probe in the shell. Some instruments which are specifically designed for the immersion technique may have gates that track, or stay attached to the echoes, even if the pattern moves left or right on the screen.

Remember that there will be a slightly different pattern from an immersion scan than from an applanation scan. In the immersion technique, you should expect to be able to see a double echo from the cornea. As mentioned earlier, the double echo is produced by the anterior and posterior surfaces of the cornea. This separation of the corneal echoes is not apparent in the applanation technique due to the large echo from the probe tip merging with the echoes from the cornea.

Always look for the corneal double peak when using the immersion technique. It is a common mistake to see the echo from the anterior lens, which sometimes appears first, and think that it is the corneal echo. Watch for the anterior segment pattern of three echoes. These three are the double-peaked corneal echo, and the anterior and posterior lens echoes. Realize that the curvature of the cornea will make it a bit tricky to locate the echoes from the cornea because there is only one possible position of the probe which will allow the beam to be directed perpendicularly toward it. When the probe is off axis, the corneal echo will drop down very suddenly, often so far that it is not viewed on the screen. Using a scleral shell that holds the probe makes finding the corneal echo quite a bit easier, but after just a little practice, a successful scan may be obtained using any of the shell designs.

Once these anterior segment echoes are obtained, observe the echoes from the posterior segment (retina, sclera, and orbital fat). When moving the probe to improve the quality of these echoes, you may lose the anterior echoes. It requires only miniscule movements of the probe to change the echo pattern, so try to move as slowly as possible so that the effect of the probe movement may be observed before trying another position.

Although the immersion technique is somewhat more challenging to learn, it provides such reproducible results that it can actually take less time to perform than applanation. You might well ask, How can that be? Numerous echographers have reported that once the technique becomes routine, patients are in and out of the examining chair in as little as five to ten minutes, a time comparable to that of the applanation method. These echographers feel that scans are repeated more frequently with the contact technique because of the need to continually ascertain that there is not too much pressure on the cornea.

SLIT LAMP APPLANATION

The slit lamp method for performing A-scans is the most commonly used technique today. The patient is seated at the slit lamp or chin rest and no gel or scleral shell is required. However, if you think carefully about the idea of a hard probe tip touching a cornea, the problem of corneal compression may be appreciated. Reducing this decidedly negative factor is possible, and will be covered in the sections that follow.

A perfectly balanced slit lamp or chin rest is essential to success with biometry. Make sure the carriage mechanism moves freely so as to avoid any undue movements near or on a patient's cornea.

The advantages of using a slit lamp are:

1. No additional equipment purchase is required.
2. The patient is already accustomed to sitting at the slit lamp.
3. The technique is very similar to applanation tonometry.
4. The joy stick control allows for minute probe changes.

The disadvantages of using a slit lamp are:

1. Performing A-scans can tie up that exam lane.
2. Care must be taken when using a tonometer mount to avoid damage to the tonometer.
3. Care must be taken to correctly balance the tonometer for optimal corneal contact pressure.
4. It is difficult to position wheelchair patients at a slit lamp.

Equipment

The slit lamp applanation technique may be performed with either one of two setups. The most common method is to utilize the existing slit lamp in one of the examining lanes. The second method uses a KOWA chin rest with a special probe mount.

Tonometer

The slit lamp must have a Goldman-type tonometer in which to mount the probe, or it may be fitted with a mounting adaptor obtained from the ultrasound instrument company. When using the tonometer, the probe will have to be carefully balanced so that minimal pressure is applied to the cornea.

There is a routine for determining the appropriate setting on the tonometer. A knob on the side of the tonometer is adjusted during use. The setting will vary depending upon the type of probe. It is more important to understand how to balance any tonometer than to simply memorize a preset value.

First, the probe must be mounted into the tonometer. If the prism is still in place, gently remove it by pulling it out from the patient side while supporting the mechanism. Insert the A-scan probe from the back. There may be a very tiny screw on the back of the ring which holds the prism. The purpose of this screw is to make it impossible to insert the prism from the wrong direction. Unfortunately, it also prevents the A-scan probe from being positioned as well. Therefore, use a jeweler's screwdriver to remove the screw. There is no real need to replace it.

Once the probe is positioned in the tonometer ring, secure the cord by looping a rubber band around the wire, then around some part of the slit lamp. This serves several purposes. It will support the weight of the cable, making balancing of the tonometer easier, and in the event of an unexpected tug on the wire, the elasticity now provided will offer protection for the cord's connection points on the probe and the tonometer itself, and reduces unnecessary movements of the probe near the patient's eye.

Now that the probe is correctly positioned, turn the tonometer knob to zero and gently touch the probe tip with a sterile cotton-tipped applicator. This simulates the type of contact that will be made with the cornea. Notice the stiffness and the way in which the probe returns to its original position when you let go.

Begin to slowly turn the tonometer knob to a higher number. Watch the probe carefully and observe at what point the whole probe assembly shifts its weight forward.

Again, gently push on the tip and let go. The probe

should move forward to its resting position after you release the pressure on the tip. If the probe is still resting in a tilted back position, then turn the tonometer knob to a slightly higher value.

The ultimate goal is to adjust the pressure on the tonometer to such a point where a gentle yet constant pressure will be applied to the cornea. There is no magic number for this setting. It is important to set the tonometer pressure each day the slit lamp is to be used for axial eye length measurements. This will ensure that the smallest possible pressure will be exerted on the cornea. As with all axial length procedures, gentle use of the joy stick on the slit lamp is an important factor in reducing corneal compression.

When the A-scans are completed, replace the tonometer prism and check to make sure that the orientation marks on the prism are aligned with the marks on the ring.

Chin Rest

Most manufactures of ultrasound equipment offer a free-standing chin rest, often made by KOWA, which has a probe mounting adaptor. This chin rest provides what the echographer needs with respect to positioning the patient and moving the A-scan probe to the eye.

The same careful treatment of the wire from the probe should be given here as well. Tie a rubber band on the cable, then loop the other end of the elastic around the large mounting screw on the chin rest. There is no knob

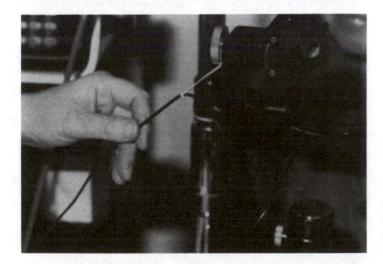

Figure 4.31 To minimize negative effects from an accidental pull on the wire, secure it with a rubber band.

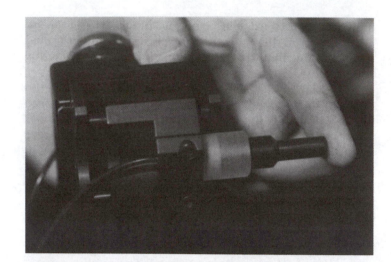

Figure 4.32 *Prior to disinfecting, test the pressure exerted by the probe tip. Rebalance if necessary.*

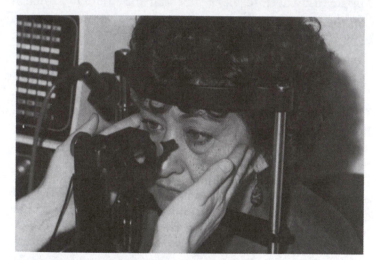

Figure 4.33 *Position patient squarely at the chin rest.*

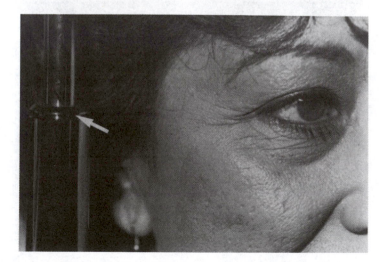

Figure 4.34 *Align marker on slit lamp with outer canthus.*

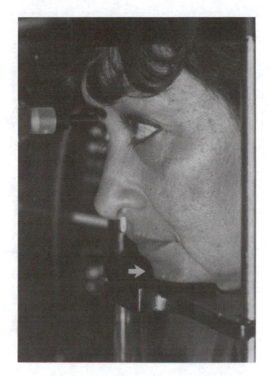

Figure 4.35 Incorrect position—chin back.

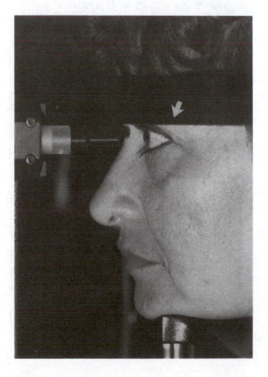

Figure 4.36 Incorrect position—forehead band low.

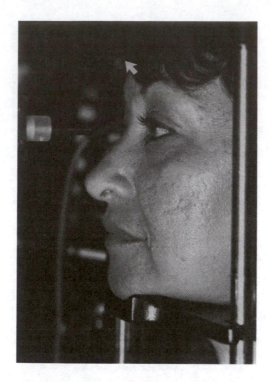

Figure 4.37 Incorrect position—forehead not touching band.

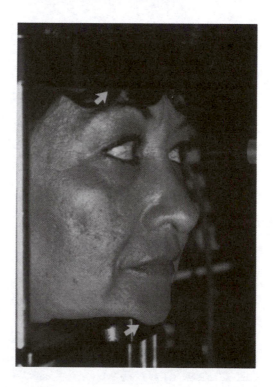

Figure 4.38 Correct position of patient and probe is out of eyelash range. The patient may freely blink during alignment process.

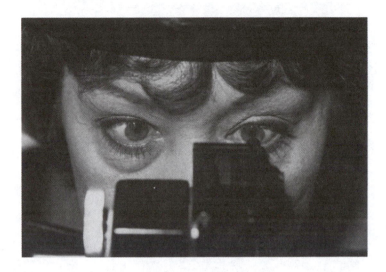

Figure 4.39 *Often patients converge when looking at the probe's fixation light, increasing difficulty of alignment.*

to balance the probe assembly. Generally, the mounting adaptors offered by the ultrasound companies exert a light pressure on the cornea.

It is important, however, to verify that the adaptor is in fact giving the gentle pressure desired. Always check it in the same way as the tonometer-mounted probes by touching the probe tip with a sterile applicator. Unfortunately, I have found old adaptors that were rusted in a fixed position, and the echographer was having a terrible time with nonreproducible measurements. Each time the probe touched the eye, the cornea was compressed giving wildly varying axial length values and confusing the technician.

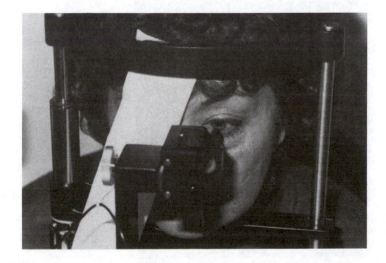

Figure 4.40 *Occluding fellow eye greatly enhances the ability to fixate and to keep the forehead tight on the band as the patient is instructed not to let the tissue fall.*

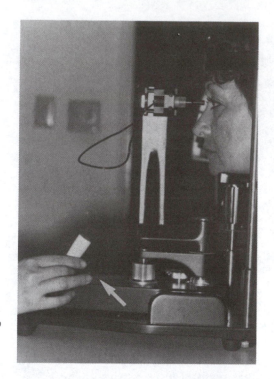

Figure 4.41 Incorrect forward position of joy stick on slit lamp produces poor maneuverability of probe toward and onto cornea.

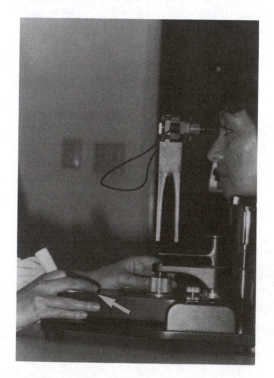

Figure 4.42 Correct position of joy stick is to be held back during alignment allowing more delicate probe movements toward and onto cornea.

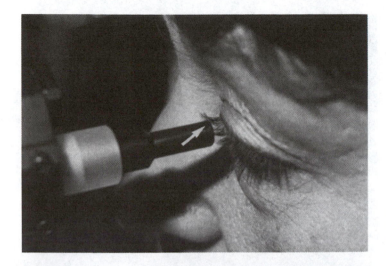

Figure 4.43 Avoid eyelashes touching probe tip. It is unsanitary and disturbing to patient.

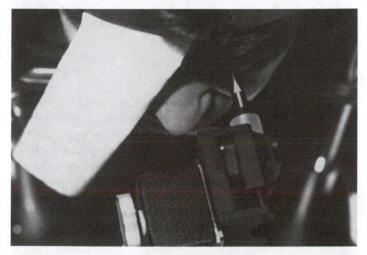

Figure 4.44 To avoid off angle probe positioning, stand up to view the angle at which the sound beam enters the eye. Probe is incorrectly directed nasally.

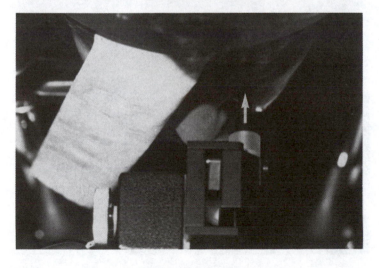

Figure 4.45 Correct alignment of probe is perpendicular to the plane of the face, with sound beam through the center of the pupil toward the macula.

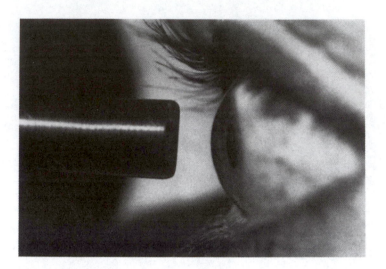

Figure 4.46 Patient has just blinked and probe is slowly moved toward cornea.

Replacing the adaptor with a new, lightly balanced one solved the problem.

Preparing the Instrument

When using an older unit without freeze frame, the instrument will have to be adjusted in order to set the correct magnification and left/right positioning of the image on the screen. There are different ways to set up an instrument depending on whether the probe is fluid-filled or solid. Be sure that the proper velocities are set for the type of eye to be measured.

In the newer digital units, the magnification and horizontal positioning are automatically set by the internal pro-

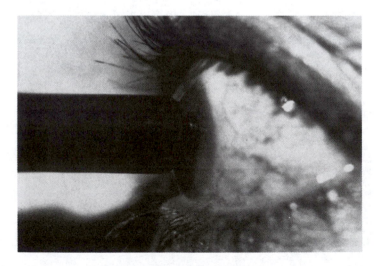

Figure 4.47 Solid A-scan probe is gently in contact with the tear film of cornea.

gram. Clean the probe as outlined earlier. If the probe is filled with distilled water, check for air bubbles and inspect the condition of the membrane on the tip.

Preparing the Patient

After instilling the anesthetic drop, position the patient comfortably at the slit lamp. Check the position of the forehead band with respect to the patient's brow. The band should be centered across the forehead. Next check the chin position. Ask the patient to place their chin as far forward as is comfortable. This will reduce head movements. Make sure that their head rests squarely on the chin rest, and that they are not tilting their head in any direction.

Now ask the patient if they are comfortable and observe their position, paying close attention to their neck. If they seem to be reaching up to keep their forehead on the band, lower the slit lamp table slightly. In this way, they will be able to hold their head up against the band.

Three of the most common problems when performing applanation A-scans can be solved in one simple way. The first problem is that patients converge (turn their eyes in) when trying to fixate on the probe's light. The second is that they can't see the fixation target. The third is that patients back away from the forehead band, making A-scans a cat and mouse game of chasing after the eye. All of these can be readily corrected by occluding the eye not being measured. The simplest method I have seen involves the use of a tissue.

A tissue folded lengthwise is placed between the patient's forehead and the slit lamp band in order to cover the non-measured eye. With the tissue draped at an angle alongside the nose there are three major benefits:

1. Occlusion of the fellow eye prevents convergence.
2. Occlusion of the fellow eye allows the fixation light inside the probe to be more easily seen.
3. If the patient backs away during the exam, the tissue falls and the examiner can stop chasing the eye and reposition the patient correctly.

In general, there will be as much if not more time spent in properly positioning the patient and caring for the equipment as is spent actually scanning.

Thoughts While Performing Applanation

Preventing corneal compression is probably the most important concern during applanation. Once the proper

Be a "cornea monitor." Keep a mental stopwatch going and get the probe off the cornea if a scan is taking too long. Always be aware of the position of both the probe and patient.

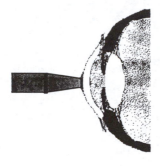

Figure 4.48 Correct applanation pressure to cornea—probe tip is in gentle contact with the cornea.

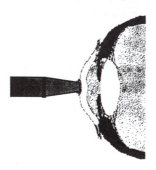

Figure 4.49 Too much applanation pressure compresses the cornea, producing falsely shallow anterior chamber depth and falsely short axial length.

adjustments have been made to ensure a gentle touch, concentrate next on the alignment of the probe. As discussed in the section on immersion scans, it helps to imagine the invisible ultrasound beam as being a tiny narrow beam of light.

The beam must be directed through the center of the cornea and lens and perpendicularly toward the macula. When preparing to perform an applanation, most of the alignment can be made long before the probe ever touches an eye. Only small movements of the probe should take place once the cornea is applanated.

When the patient and the probe are positioned, check to see that the screen of the instrument and its controls are within easy reach. Place the instrument as close to the patient's head as possible so that there is a minimum of movement on your part in glancing back and forth between the patient and the screen. One last caution: have the foot switch ready and be poised over it if that is the method by which you store a scan or take a picture. Once the probe is in contact with the eye, it is not a good idea to go looking for the foot switch.

Hold the joy stick all the way back and keep it there while slowly moving the slit lamp closer to the patient. Stop when the probe is about one-half inch from the ends of the eyelashes. I call this "keeping the probe just out of eyelash range." During the time spent aligning the probe, the patient's lashes should not come in contact with the tip. There are three reasons for keeping the probe away from the lashes:

1. It is unpleasant for the patient to feel the probe so close to their eye.
2. It is potentially both unsanitary and unsafe as material from the lashes, make-up for example, could adhere to the probe tip and then be transferred to the cornea.
3. During the probe alignment period, the patient may freely blink and therefore be more comfortable.

With the probe in this position, examine its direction. Is it perpendicular to the cornea? Is it centered over the pupil? With the room lights turned down low enough, it is often possible to see the reflection of the A-scan probe's internal light in the patient's cornea. This is helpful in aiming the sound beam through the central cornea.

Look around the slit lamp from the side and judge its position relative to the center of the cornea. Then stand up and look down with a "bird's-eye view" to judge the angle of the probe. Is it pointed nasally? Temporally? Is it directed toward the macula? Checking the probe alignment from various perspectives will greatly increase your ability to obtain valid A-scan images quickly.

When the probe is aligned and ready to make contact with the cornea, instruct the patient to "blink a couple of times and open wide." Immediately move the probe forward with the joy stick. Once the probe is in contact with the tear film of the cornea, there should be movement of echoes on the display screen. Observe the echo pattern and quickly determine which echoes need improvement.

Since the posterior lens echo is often a bit lower than the anterior capsule echo, don't worry as much about trying to make it a hundred percent tall. Begin by focusing your attention on the retinal echo, evaluating its leading edge. Is the edge smooth or coarse? Next, look for the sclera and a few orbital signals. When the retinal pattern is observed, double-check the lens echoes. It may be necessary to adjust the orientation of the probe slightly. A series of small probe movements will produce the classic A-scan echogram.

Keep a mental stopwatch running so that the probe does not stay on the eye too long. Ten to 15 seconds is a maximum time to scan, after which if there is no scan worth freezing, pull back on the joy stick and tell the patient to blink. If you feel that you may have kept the probe on the cornea a bit longer than desired, have the patient close their eyes for 10 seconds. Before beginning the next scan, always have the patient blink immediately prior to applanation. It is the duty of the examiner to maintain the moisture level of the cornea.

Remember that if only one echo appears from the back of the eye, the sound beam is directed toward the optic disk, not the macula. The macular region is slightly temporal to the disk, so look at the angle of the probe. Redirect it a bit more temporally. There should then be a scleral signal to the right of the retinal echo. The macula is the most important part of the retina and is where the most desirable echo pattern is produced.

With some patients, there may not be a significant difference in measured axial length between scans made to the disk and scans made to the macula. However, with other patients there is a huge difference, sometimes as much as 2 mm between readings on the same eye. This potential mismatch is the most important reason for confirming sound beam alignment to the macula.

It is an interesting observation that the scan often improves dramatically when the probe is moved slightly nasally and slightly superior to the point where the examiner assumes the center of the cornea to be. However, in the event that

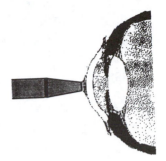

Figure 4.50 Too little applanation pressure—fluid bridge between probe tip and cornea causes falsely deep anterior chamber depth and falsely long axial length.

Once contact with the cornea is made and a good scan is displayed, resist the temptation to freeze it immediately. Pull the probe straight back until the echo pattern disappears, then immediately return to the cornea. Always check for corneal compression. Even the most experienced echographers check carefully with each and every scan.

no probe position produces a valid echo pattern on the screen, report these unusual findings to the surgeon. He may suggest a pathological condition that may have hindered your ability to obtain a valid A-scan. As mentioned earlier, staphyloma is one such condition. Pre-retinal membranes, tumor, or detachment are other possible conditions. If located along the visual axis, these may be detected on the axial length scan.

Not all patients are scanable. By that I mean that there are compromises to be made when the eye will not produce an optimal echo pattern. Sometimes a less than desirable A-scan pattern must be accepted as it is the only scan you can obtain.

Before the discussion of manual versus automatic freezing of optimal A-scan patterns, there is one vital question about technique to be answered: How do you know if you are pushing too hard on the cornea? Once the probe touches the cornea and a valid scan is displayed, gently pull the probe off the tear film. The image will disappear from the screen. Immediately go forward again with the joy stick until contact is just made and freeze the scan. You may be using a unit which does not freeze the actual echoes; such units usually have a foot switch that will at least freeze the measurement.

By "pulling off" the eye and immediately returning the probe to the cornea, the gentlest touch may be made, thereby increasing the accuracy of the measurement.

HAND-HELD APPLANATION

Hand-held applanation is mentioned last on the list of desirable methods for a variety of reasons. First, however, let me say that there are those for whom this is an appropriate method because it produces good results for them. Also, there are patients for whom this may be the only possible examination technique due to a coexistent condition. Additionally, technical advancements are being made with respect to how the hand-held probe may be designed to minimize corneal compression.

The fundamental problem with this technique is that the human hand cannot make the fine, independent movements of a slit lamp mechanism. Therefore, when the probe needs to be moved nasally, how do you know that you are not also moving it vertically or even pressing harder? All of these questions must be considered by the examiner in order to obtain as accurate a measurement as possible.

All of the previously discussed points regarding slit lamp applanation apply to the hand-held method. Comfortable positions for both the patient and the examiner will promote success.

AUTOMATIC VERSUS MANUAL FREEZING

This section deals with those digital instruments that have the ability to freeze the A-scan on the screen. This is probably the single most beneficial advancement made in this field in many years. Although instruments may have many "bells and whistles," their most important function is to provide a clear image of the echogram for the examiner to evaluate. This frozen image may be created in two ways:

Practice with manual and automatic modes of acquiring an A-scan. Know how they work so that when necessary the modes can be switched to see if that improves the ability to get a reading.

1. Manually, the examiner may depress a foot switch when the desired echo pattern appears on the screen.
2. The instrument may be "intelligent" and freeze the image automatically when it "thinks" it sees a valid scan.

Manual Freeze

Manual freeze is the mode I generally select. The reason for this is that I want to have full control over which scan is chosen. After making initial contact with the cornea, I want to be able to pull the probe off, put it back on, then freeze. I feel that this gives me the chance to actively scan the eye, observing the relative quality of echoes. It also provides the opportunity to move the probe off, then on to check for compression.

Auto Freeze

Most newer axial length instruments have a mode which automatically freezes the A-scan and produces a measurement. And there are certainly cases for which this can be helpful. A highly uncooperative patient is one such case. If the patient cannot or will not hold still for you, then this mode can be a blessing. However, the ability of the instrument to freeze a truly valid scan is only as good as the ability of the person who wrote the computer program. The qualities of a valid scan that are programmed into an A-scan unit are called algorithms. This word appears frequently in discussions of "intelligent" computers. The algorithms are what determine which scan will be accepted for auto freeze and which scans will not.

Not all eyes are scanable. Some have retinal problems that make obtaining a classic retinal echo impossible. If the patient has a staphyloma for example, try the immersion technique.

I feel very strongly that there is no A-scan system available which is smarter than the operator who uses it. Also, no A-scan unit available should be operated by an individual who does not understand the principles of ultrasound and what constitutes a valid echogram.

Use the auto-freeze mode with the understanding that you must agree with the instrument's determination of a scan's validity. If you do not agree, repeat the scan. As mentioned earlier, all available methods and modes should be tried so that each patient will have their needs met.

CONCLUDING REMARKS

There is certainly a lot to learn about performing axial length measurements. And there are still opportunities for increasing your knowledge even after you have mastered the techniques themselves. It is quite useful and satisfying to understand why a patient's scan looks the way it does or why those wild measurements are correct for that individual. What makes the difference between simply approaching the procedure as a routine task and really understanding what is going on is taking the time to think things through and to seek advice about puzzling cases. With perseverance and a willingness to search for answers to questions, you will not only become confident that the best has been provided for your patients, but soon you will be the one who is asked for advice about difficult scans.

CHAPTER 5

Corneal Thickness Pachymetry

CORNEAL THICKNESS

Measuring the thickness of the cornea is another form of biometry. The corneal specialist may have many reasons for wanting to know this parameter. Refractive surgery and corneal grafts are probably the most common. In this biometric procedure, called pachymetry, corneal measurements are not given in millimeters as in axial length, but are recorded in microns. There are 1,000 microns in a millimeter (and 1,000 millimeters in a meter). Therefore, an average cornea which is said to measure 500 microns is one-half of one millimeter thick. This value could be written as 500 microns or 0.5 millimeter. Generally, an instrument specifically designed for this type of measurement will display the measured values in microns.

BASIC PRINCIPLES REVISITED

The principles of ultrasonography apply in the same way for the corneal scan as for any other type of scanning. The sound beam must be perpendicular to both the anterior and posterior surfaces of the cornea. This is a relatively easy task in the center of the cornea, but it becomes more difficult at the periphery. This is because in the center of the cornea, the anterior and posterior surfaces are parallel to each other. At the periphery, however, they are no longer parallel, making it more difficult to align the sound beam appropriately to both surfaces.

All the same principles needed to perform an axial length measurement apply to the cornea as well. With the cornea, however, there are only two echoes with which to be concerned, the anterior and posterior corneal surfaces.

SPECIAL THOUGHTS ABOUT THE CORNEA

Just as in axial length scans, we must pay great respect to the patient's cornea. Keeping the probe on the eye for the minimum amount of time is a key goal. Also, any time the patient is not being scanned, ask them to close their eyes so that the corneas do not dry out. A topical anesthetic can

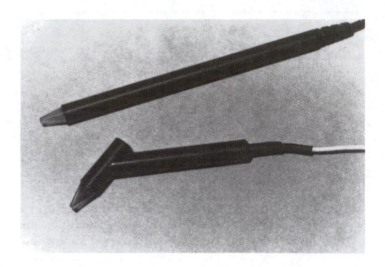

Figure 5.1 Two different pachymetry probes, straight and angled tips.

reduce the patient's urge to blink, which of course is helpful for scanning, but be careful to encourage blinking and thereby keep the cornea moist.

PREPARING THE INSTRUMENT

It is common to have a separate instrument for performing pachymetry, although some systems have multiple modalities. One thing for certain is that the probe for measuring the cornea will be different from the one for measuring axial length.

Another fundamental difference is the velocity of sound for the cornea. This value can range from 1600 m/s to 1640 m/s. Although the accepted velocity values for axial length measurements are fairly universal, the values for the cornea vary slightly. A velocity of 1620 m/s is a well-accepted median value. Note which velocity is being used in your instrument. If the values are user programmable, be certain that the sound speed remains the same from one patient to the next.

Clean the pachymetry probe in the same way solid biometry probes are cleaned. Position the screen near the patient's head and have the foot switch ready. (See the section in chapter 4 describing sterilization procedures.)

Position yourself so that you do not have to move anything but your eyes to see both the patient's cornea and the screen of the instrument.

PREPARING THE PATIENT

Instill a topical anesthetic in the normal manner. Try to provide some sort of fixation target for the patient such as a movable light or marks on the ceiling. Be certain that the patient is comfortably reclined and that you are comfortably seated so that both of you will be relaxed.

TECHNIQUES

Although each physician may request a different series of measurements, the most common measurement is the central corneal thickness. When this is included in a series, begin with it for several reasons. First of all, the center of the cornea is the easiest area to measure since the two corneal surfaces are very nearly parallel at this location. Secondly, this will typically be the thinnest part of the cornea and the measured value can be useful when judging the validity of data from other parts of the cornea. Occasionally, there may be an area of the peripheral cornea which is thinner than the central reading, but this is quite unusual.

There are two fundamental methods for mapping the thickness of various parts of the cornea. One way is to start in the center and measure along the same radius out to the periphery. The measurements should start out small and then gradually increase as you move more peripherally.

The second method is to measure one "ring" at a time. This means that imaginary concentric rings on the cornea are used as guides in placing the probe for measurements. The first ring is 3 mm in diameter and is located in the center of the cornea. The next ring is usually 6 or 7 mm in diameter, and larger rings may be measured as well. Measurements from the first ring are the most critical for radial keratometry procedures since this is the area in which the incisions are started.

Sometimes measuring corneal thickness by radius is a bit easier. Changing the probe's angle for each corneal position takes conscious thought with regard to maintaining perpendicularity.

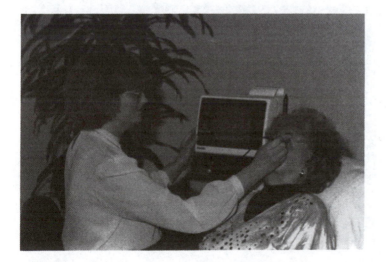

Figure 5.2 Positioning of the patient's head near the instrument is an important part of good technique.

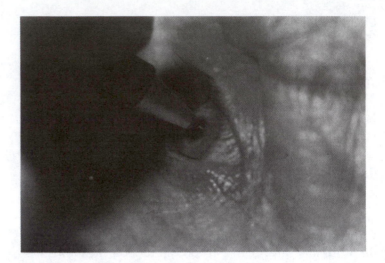

Figure 5.3 Central corneal thickness is being measured. Note that the angle of the probe is perpendicular to both corneal surfaces.

The advantage of this method is that the examiner may notice an area of corneal thinning more easily. When measuring parts of the cornea that are all the same distance from the center, there should be close agreement between the values.

For every measurement, the examiner must imagine the path of the sound beam and align the probe perpendicular to both surfaces of the cornea. If the probe were aligned obliquely, then the echo from the posterior surface of the cornea would probably not be tall enough on the screen to be measured; and if it were in fact tall enough to be measured, then the measurement would be too long. A valid

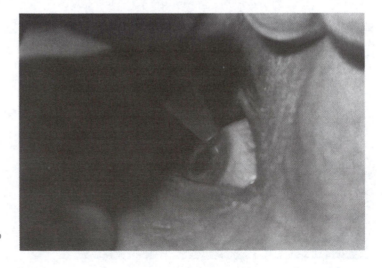

Figure 5.4 Peripheral corneal measurement being made. Note the different probe angle from the central reading. The sound beam is perpendicular to the peripheral corneal surfaces.

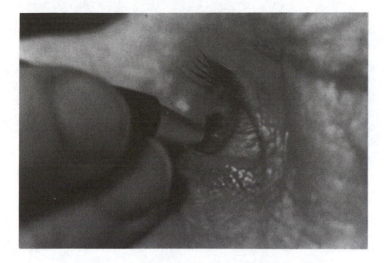

Figure 5.5 Off axis peripheral corneal scan probably produces no measurement or a falsely long one. The probe is not perpendicular to the corneal surfaces.

pachymetry reading is the smallest reproducible value which would indicate perpendicularity with both surfaces.

Unfortunately, most pachymetry instruments do not provide the examiner with an echogram from which to make a judgment. This can be frustrating, for when the numbers come up on the screen, there is no way of confirming the quality of the echo pattern that produced them. Such instruments rely entirely on the internal algorithms mentioned before. We can only assume that the computer programmer did a good job in deciding what the instrument should accept as a valid scan. This can account for the fact that some instruments work differently from others in the way they behave when producing a measurement.

Another problem resulting from not being able to see the echoes is that the gain could be turned up so high that reverberation artifacts might interfere with the measurement.

The average corneal thickness is about 500 microns, or one-half of a millimeter.

CONCLUDING REMARKS

The pachymetry part of ophthalmic echography is not utilized as much as axial length A-scans or diagnostic B-scans. This is probably due in part to the fact that the cornea, being so easy to examine, usually does not require sophisticated instrumentation to evaluate its condition.

With consideration given to thoroughly understanding how your instrument makes its decisions as to what constitutes a valid corneal reading, positive results may be obtained. A good deal of common sense is called for in this procedure as well as in the other forms of ultrasound, since we have to make our own evaluations of measurements based on logic. For example, if the central corneal measurement is 524 microns, then it would be illogical for a peripheral reading to be 496 microns. Also, a central measurement of less than 500 microns would be considered a thin cornea, whereas a reading of greater than 600 microns indicates a thick cornea. Remember that when measuring close to the limbus, values can increase more quickly and several readings must be taken before a level of confidence is achieved.

CHAPTER 6

Diagnostic B-scan

DIAGNOSTIC B-SCAN

B-scans are two-dimensional ultrasound images created by lighted dots of varying brightness. This may sound somewhat abstract, but in chapter 1, we learned that the B in B-scan stands for brightness. The varying levels of brightness on a B-scan echogram can provide the examiner with a wealth of information about the tissues that produced them.

Unlike the A-scan, a B-scan image has curved parts. I'll be honest with you, the first time I looked at a B-scan back in 1978, all I could relate to was the fact that there was a curved echo pattern on the screen, and eyeballs were round. Learning how to interpret B-scan images takes time and, as might be expected, lots of patience.

INDICATIONS

Since a B-scan shows the geometry and geography of ocular structures, it is a useful tool for observing things that cannot be seen in any other way. The most obvious example is a vitreous hemorrhage. Not only can the patient not see out of the eye, but the physician cannot see in. In this instance, a B-scan will provide a map of the eye and orbit allowing the physician to select the most appropriate method for managing the condition. Even in the case of a cataract, if the fundus is not clearly visible, a B-scan would provide valuable information about the physical condition of the retina and the contour of the globe. Another case that would warrant a B-scan preoperatively is the patient with a staphyloma. Every now and then when a patient is given a retrobulbar injection prior to surgery, the needle accidentally punctures the globe. Sometimes this can be due to an irregularly shaped eye and an inability to obtain an understanding of the boundaries of this staphyloma. It has been recommended that a preoperative B-scan be made in preparation for giving a retrobulbar injection in such abnormally contoured globes.

Any time a clear view of the retina is not possible, a B-scan is indicated. Know the history of the patient so that an appropriate examination method may be chosen. A patient with a foreign body may have had a perforation of the globe and a very low intraocular pressure. When in doubt, consult the physician, as this may change the examination technique.

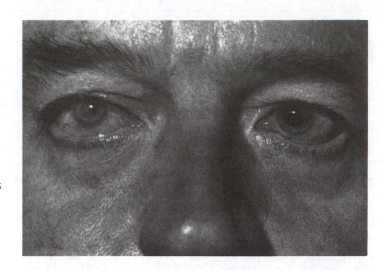

Figure 6.1 When a patient has an opaque media such as a scarred cornea, the B-scan is a very useful tool for imaging parts of the eye not visible to the ophthalmologist.

Even when the ocular media are clear, a B-scan can add information to that obtained with an ophthalmoscope. For example, if one eye protrudes more than the other or is **displaced** from the normal position, a B-scan can be an effective method of screening the extraocular muscles and orbit. Many things could be causing the proptosis, such as enlarged muscles or even a mass behind or to the side of the globe.

Foreign bodies are another indication for a B-scan. Determining the presence of a foreign body and its relationship to ocular structures is an important part of the workup in such cases. X-ray, CT, or MRI can be used as well to help determine the material of which the foreign body is made and to help in discerning whether the object is inside or outside the globe. In trauma cases, the B-scan is often the quickest and easiest method of determining the status of the globe.

In addition to topographical information, the B-scan can also provide information about the consistency of the structures being imaged. The internal structure of tumors, for example, can be quite different from one type to another. Looking at histology slides of various types of tumor cells and thinking about the basic ultrasound principles can help the examiner make educated judgments about possible diagnoses. Even the B-scan probe itself can be used to consciously apply a bit of pressure to the globe while an orbital tumor image is shown. This will help to determine if the mass is compressible. The compressibility of a lesion is another clue in making a diagnosis.

GETTING STARTED

Every little bit that you learn while performing B-scans builds up your mental reference library. Slowly but surely, images fall into place in your mind; it will be like having keys to unlock more mysteries than you can imagine. This chapter will introduce the basic scanning techniques and will help you gain a better understanding of what the images mean.

The Role of the Technician

The purpose of this chapter is not to teach technicians to diagnose disease. That would not be correct. The diagnosis is technically made by the physician. However, the technician can be an extremely valuable member of the diagnostic team.

A thorough understanding of the anatomy, physiology, and pathology of the eye is essential for the conscientious ophthalmic echographer. You need to have access to clinical information in order to understand the disease processes of ocular conditions. The role of the technician certainly includes being able to effectively scan all parts of the globe and orbit for evidence of pathology. Being able to confidently make a suggestion as to the actual diagnosis comes much later, after many, many scans have been performed and understood.

The First Scan

Begin at the beginning by scanning yourself. Assuming that your eye is average, you will be able to really see how a globe's curvature should appear and how the optic nerve is imaged. With the picture of a normal eye permanently engraved in your memory, when an abnormal image appears you will be instantly alerted. Watching the screen while scanning your own eye also offers an increased appreciation for how a tiny probe movement can make a big change in the image.

Look at the patient. Are their eyes the same? Make some observations prior to performing a B-scan. Make certain that any obvious clues do not go unnoticed.

Learning From Known Pathologies

Next, scan clear media cases. That is, scan patients whose pathology is clearly visible to both you and the physician. In this way the ultrasound images can be studied while you have a sharp mental image of the actual location, size, and shape of the pathology.

Every time you perform a B-scan, you are adding more mental images to your reference library. Hundreds of scans must be performed in order to build up that source of clinical information.

Test yourself by visualizing what the image will look like on the screen prior to placing the probe on the eye. If you have a clear understanding, you will be right most of the time. If you find yourself looking at an image that wasn't expected, figure out where it came from and learn why it appeared. Ask yourself these questions: "In what direction was the patient looking?" "Where was the orientation mark on the probe?" "If I put the probe here, how will the image change?" Don't be afraid to get up and walk around the room if you need to think about what you are seeing on the screen. There is no substitute for logically thinking through each examination. Take the time necessary to build confidence.

The Final Step

Know your own eye. Scan yourself so that you may judge the inherent quality of another instrument should you have to use something different. Monitoring the image in this way can also provide a signal when your own equipment may not be performing up to standard.

The final step is to scan opaque media cases, the patients for whom a B-scan will give invaluable information, guiding the physician in the best course of management.

When there is sufficient doubt in the mind of an examiner, they should not hesitate to send the patient for a second echographic opinion. Many of the country's medical schools have well-developed ophthalmic echography departments to which a patient may be referred.

EQUIPMENT AND SUPPLIES

There are a few items that make performing B-scans easier. One is an adjustable fellow eye fixation target. This is par-

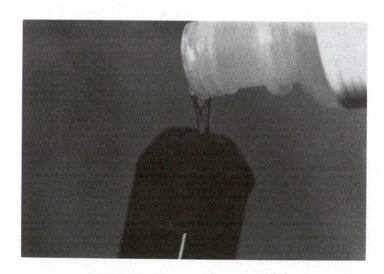

Figure 6.2 Copious amounts of sterile 2.5% methylcellulose may be applied to the probe tip, the patient's eye, or both.

ticularly important for open eye scans and will be discussed below in the section on techniques. Also, since patient comfort is very high on the list of important things to consider, I prefer an examination chair that reclines. As mentioned before, lying flat is very hard on the lower back and we want the patient to be physically comfortable.

Occasionally there may be a need to perform a mini-immersion B-scan for evaluating the anterior segment. For this special exam, a set of scleral shells is generally used. Details are covered in the techniques section below.

Most of the other materials required for a diagnostic B-scan are readily available. Make sure you have plenty of these basic items:

Store gel bottles upside down and remove the dropper tips. This will minimize air bubble problems.

1. Sterile methylcellulose 2.5% solution
2. Topical anesthetic
3. Sterile irrigating solution
4. Alcohol preps
5. Tissues
6. Photographic film

TECHNIQUES

A most important goal of any scanning technique is to peform examinations in a consistent manner. This encourages a thorough and accurate observation of all parts of the globe and orbit. There are many different ways to approach this and I will cover what I believe to be the most reliable system.

Be consistent by performing each echographic examination in the same manner, beginning with one particular probe position and moving on to others. In this way, there will not be a concern that something might have been overlooked. The fear of missing a pathology is a valid one to have. Using a systematic approach, whichever one you choose, will increase your feeling of having completed an adequate and proper examination.

In the event of an especially puzzling case, seek out someone more experienced than you to whom you can turn with a question. As you observe other echographers, learn from them and integrate into your own examination techniques those new ideas which you find useful. Some institutions have programs that will allow observers to study for a period of time, a week or month, for a fee. And even echographers who have been doing B-scans for years have told me that they have gained immeasurable knowledge while observing for two weeks in an echography department.

Unfortunately, one of the sad things overall about learning ultrasonography is that there are no schools which offer degrees in it, and only a few short courses are available here and there throughout the country. A list of organizations that may be contacted regarding available courses in ultrasound are listed in chapter 9.

Probe Orientation

Before we can begin to think about what each echo represents, we must understand how the orientation marker on the probe relates to the image on the screen. This will be fundamental in determining the actual location of a structure or pathology in the eye or the orbit.

The key point is that the marker on the probe indicates the top of the display screen. Each B-scan probe will have a marker, usually a white line near the tip. The transducer inside the probe oscillates back and forth, toward and away from this mark. As it pivots inside the probe, the transducer generates a fan of sound waves, similar to how a slit lamp produces a thin sector of light. This fan of sound is often appropriately called an acoustic section. We have to understand the direction of the movement of the transducer so that we can tell when the fan is being aimed vertically, horizontally, or any other way.

Vertical Transverse

When the white mark on the probe is directed vertically toward the patient's brow, or superiorly, the scan orienta-

Know how to image the macula quickly with the horizontal axial view and the longitudinal view. This is probably the most important bit of information for most patients. The doctor will want to know the status of this area of the retina. For the right eye, use the L 9:00 position, and use L 3:00 for the left.

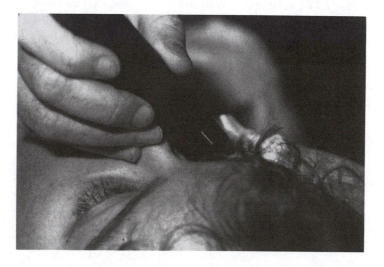

Figure 6.3 A vertical transverse scan where probe marker is superior and the probe is placed nasally to image temporally. The patient looks away from the probe.

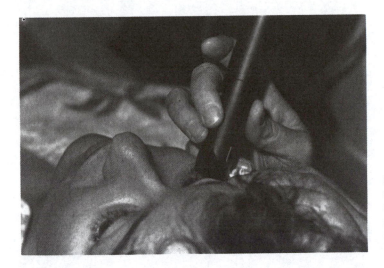

Figure 6.4 Another vertical transverse scan where probe marker is superior and the probe is placed temporally to image nasally. The patient looks away from the probe.

tion is superior/inferior. This is called a vertical transverse scan. Since the mark is up, the screen now displays a sector scan showing superior retina on the top and inferior retina on the bottom. Sounds simple enough, doesn't it?

What about the part of the scan that is in the middle of the screen? After all, the image in the center has the most resolution and this is where we want to center any unknown pathology. If the probe tip is placed on the 9:00 limbus, then the tissue directly across from the probe is at the 3:00 position. Therefore, to examine the 3:00 position in the globe, the probe is placed at 9:00. Once in the 9:00 position, the probe is shifted into the fornix so that the 3:00 meridian is scanned from **posterior to anterior**. Wherever the probe is placed on the eye, the area being scanned lies opposite.

When the probe is on the limbus, the sound beam is being directed posteriorly toward the disk. As the probe is shifted into the fornix, the scan plane moves more anteriorly. This is true for either the horizontal or vertical transverse positions.

The three main probe positions are vertical transverse, horizontal transverse, and longitudinal. All three are part of a complete echographic examination.

Horizontal Transverse

Next, let's look at the horizontal transverse scan. Convention usually calls for the orientation mark to be directed toward the nose for both the right and left eye examinations. Since the top of the screen corresponds with the mark on the probe, the top of the scan on any horizontal transverse scan is nasal retina and the bottom of the scan is temporal retina.

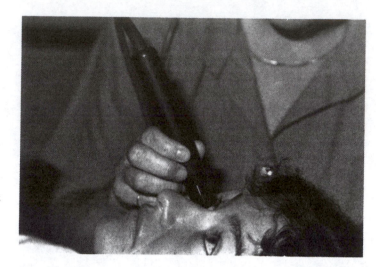

Figure 6.5 *A horizontal transverse scan; probe marker is nasal. Probe is placed at the 6:00 limbus to image 12:00 posteriorly, patient looks away from the probe.*

If the center of the probe is placed on the 6:00 limbus, for example, the center of the horizontal scan displayed will be 12:00. This meridian may then be scanned from anterior to posterior by shifting the probe from the limbus into the fornix.

The horizontal transverse scan is a particularly useful one when documenting the macula. Think of the sound beam being directed toward the optic disk when the white mark on the probe is toward the nose. The displayed scan is nasal on top, temporal on the bottom.

Now think about where the macula is in relation to the disk. It is temporal to the disk, right? If the macula is temporal to the disk and the disk is in the center of the image

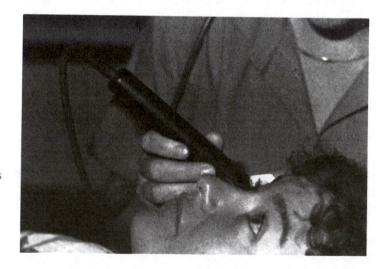

Figure 6.6 *Another horizontal transverse scan; probe marker is nasal. Probe is being moved into the inferior fornix, maintaining perpendicularity with sclera. Superior quadrant is imaged and patient looks away from the probe.*

when the temporal retina is at the bottom of the screen, then the macula will be just below the optic nerve on the image. Got it? If not, read it through again. This is an important point to understand and it is exactly the way we have to train our minds to create a mental map of the eye.

The macula can also be imaged from many other probe positions. However, having the optic nerve shadow as a point of reference makes the job much easier. A long section of the optic nerve appears on the screen as a shadow, or lack of echoes, extending posteriorly from the retina. This is due to the high reflectivity of the disk. In cross section, the optic nerve appears as a dark circle.

Oblique

Now let's look at an oblique scan angle, one that is anywhere between vertical and horizontal. In this scan, the probe may be placed on any clock hour, with the orientation mark as superior as possible. The resulting scan will be produced from the portion of the eye opposite the probe. If the probe is placed at the 7:30 position on the limbus of the left eye and the white mark is up, the top of the screen will be superonasal and the bottom of the screen will be inferotemporal. Since the probe was placed at 7:30, the center of the resulting image will be the 1:30 meridian. It really helps to have an old-fashioned clock on the wall for immediate reference.

From what you have learned about how the orientation mark determines the scan plane, any unusual scan angle may be used and understood. Just be careful to observe the position of the patient's eye in order to determine from where the image came.

Longitudinal

A longitudinal scan is created a bit differently from the basic transverse scans. The purpose of this scan position is to show the anterior/posterior extent of a structure or pathology. The other types of scans show the up/down and right/left extent of a tissue. Now we will look at the front/back extent with a longitudinal scan.

With this scan, the probe's orientation mark is always directed toward the limbus of the cornea. The transducer now swings back and forth in an anterior/posterior fashion. When creating such an image, the goal is to display the

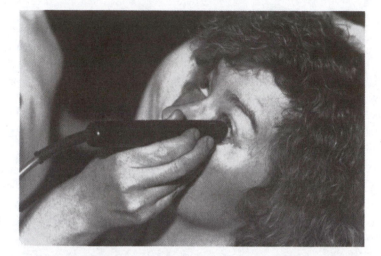

Figure 6.7 A longitudinal scan with the probe marker toward the cornea and the patient looking away. Probe is placed at the 6:00 limbus to image the 12:00 radius from optic nerve to ciliary body; image labeled L 12:00.

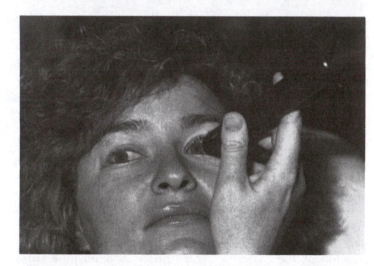

Figure 6.8 Another longitudinal scan with the probe marker toward the cornea and the patient looking away. Probe is placed at the 3:00 limbus to image the 9:00 radius from optic nerve to ciliary body; image labeled L 9:00.

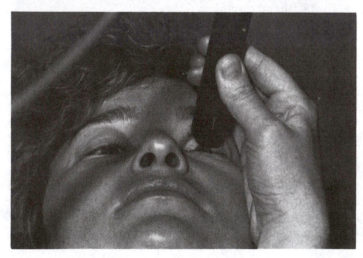

Figure 6.9 A longitudinal scan with the probe marker toward the cornea and the patient looking away. Probe is placed at the 12:00 limbus to image the 6:00 radius from optic nerve to ciliary body; image labeled L 6:00

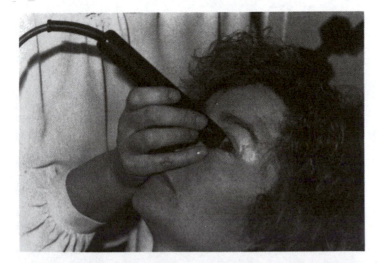

Figure 6.10 This is the most important longitudinal scan. The probe is placed at the 9:00 limbus to image the 3:00 radius of the left eye from optic nerve to ciliary body; labeled L 3:00. This probe position will image the macula. On the right eye the longitudinal macula scan is L 9:00 with the probe placed at the 3:00 limbus, marker toward cornea.

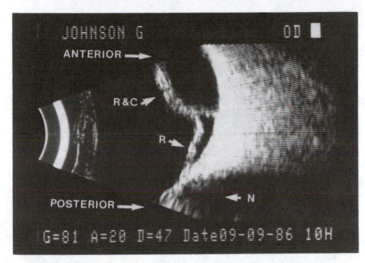

Figure 6.11 A B-scan echogram of a longitudinal scan (L 9:00) of the right eye. Optic nerve at the bottom of scan, detached retina (R) inserts at the optic disk (N) showing that the macula is off. The choroid doesn't detach until past the macula. Retina and choroid are both off (RC) farther peripherally. The top of the screen is anterior; bottom of the screen is posterior.

optic nerve shadow on the very bottom edge of the screen. The top of the scan will therefore be the ciliary body region. Slight probe movements can be made to adjust the image to show these structures.

Two of the things for which this scan is used is imaging the ciliary body and determining the anterior/posterior extent of a lesion or detachment.

Axial

The axial B-scan is one where the probe is placed directly over the cornea. The posterior lens surface and the optic nerve shadow are in the center of the image. In a vertical

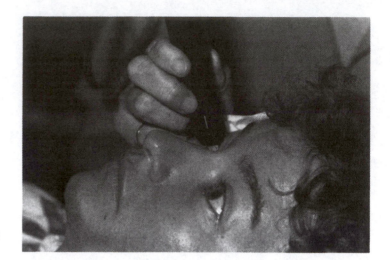

Figure 6.12 Another way to image the macula is with the horizontal axial scan. Probe mark is toward nose, patient is in primary gaze, and probe is very gently placed on the central cornea with copious gel to image visual axis.

axial view, the top of the screen is superior and the bottom of the screen is inferior. In this view, the optic nerve is visualized. The label for this scan is vertical axial even though the scan plane through the nerve is not really the visual axis of the eye since the macula is temporal to the disk. As we learned in the previous chapter, the visual axis of the eye includes the macula.

The horizontal axial scan is produced by again placing the probe over the cornea and having the marker directed toward the nose. This horizontal transverse scan plane shows the macula in relation to the optic nerve.

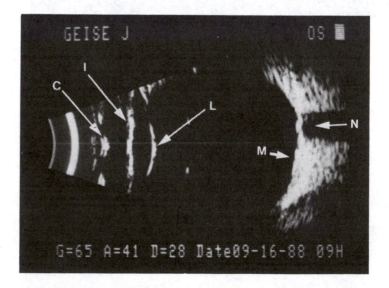

Figure 6.13 A B-scan echogram of the previous photo shows double cornea echo (C), iris (I), posterior lens (L), macula (M), optic nerve (N). Proper label is HAX which stands for horizontal axial.

The difference between axial scans and the other transverse scans is that the axial scan is directed through the central cornea and lens. All other B-scans are performed so as to carefully avoid sending the sound beam through the lens unless it is the lens itself which is being studied.

Changes in the velocity and refraction of the sound beam make it inappropriate to make judgments about the area of the retina which lies behind the imaged lens. Clinical evaluations of the retina are never made when scanning through the lens. They are made by using the various transverse and longitudinal scan angles.

The main purpose of axial scans is to provide an image with recognizable landmarks in the area of the visual axis. That is why I stated earlier that the horizontal scan plane can be particularly useful since it images the macula.

Three-Dimensional Thinking

With the probe orientation in mind, the next concept to tackle is that of thinking three-dimensionally. You will find yourself constantly asking the question, "What three-dimensional object could have produced this two-dimensional B-scan image?"

Consider a familiar three-dimensional object such as an apple. If a vertical slice is made through the center, the whole length of the core can be seen. The slice has an overall round appearance, with a vertical dark structure that runs the entire length from top to bottom.

However, take a horizontal slice through the center of that same apple and the image will be entirely different.

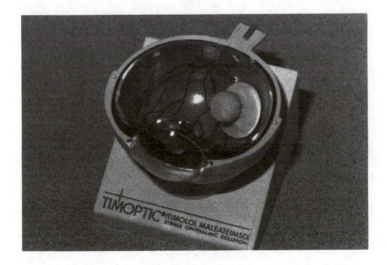

Figure 6.14 This clever idea of using clay to simulate the location of a tumor greatly assists the examiner in determining why scan images look the way they do. One can think, "If I put the probe here, what will the picture look like?" Courtesy of Lois Hart, RDMS Massachusetts Eye and Ear Infirmary, Boston.

The only thing the two images have in common is that they are round and they both come from an apple. The horizontal slice will have only one small dark structure in the center from the core.

It is the job of the echographer to create mental images of three-dimensional forms with only two-dimensional slices as guides. As will be seen, complicated pathological conditions can create a real jigsaw of images which have to be reconstructed three-dimensionally in the mind of the examiner.

Methods of Performing Scans

For well over ten years now, the majority of B-scans have been performed with a probe placed in contact with the eye, whether through closed lids or directly on the globe. This is called a contact scan. The two types of immersion scans, the mini-immersion and the water bath technique, will also be discussed in the following sections. There are times when both contact and immersion scans may be required in order to produce the best information about a patient's condition. One such condition is a ciliary body melanoma.

Closed Eye Contact Scans

For years, the majority of echographers have performed their ultrasound exams with the patient's eyes closed. A copious amount of ultrasound coupling gel was placed on the closed lid and the B-scan probe was moved to different

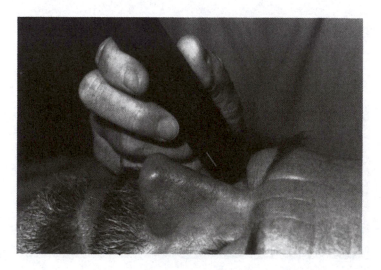

Figure 6.15 Horizontal transverse scan on closed lid with copious gel, probe directed posteriorly.

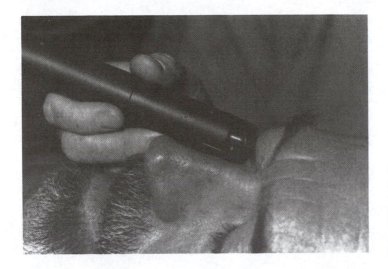

Figure 6.16 Probe being moved down into the fornix while maintaining perpendicular contact, area being imaged is superior and anterior, patient is instructed to look up.

positions while the patient was asked to look in different directions. This is considered a safe method since no corneal contact is made. However safe it may be, this method has one fundamental shortcoming. The fact is, the examiner never really knows the exact direction of the patient's gaze. This in turn makes localization of the pathology more challenging.

To understand what the patient is experiencing, try this experiment. Close your eyes and look straight ahead. With the eyes still closed, look to the right; look down and right; look straight down; look down and left; look to the left. You can imagine how tedious this can be for the patient, especially if they are nervous about losing their vision.

Be aware that if you perform closed eye B-scans, you run the risk of not knowing the direction of the patient's gaze. Patients often have a hard time trying to look in a certain direction when their eyes are closed.

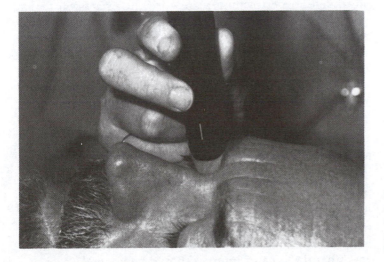

Figure 6.17 Patient looks down with probe on upper lid imaging inferiorly and posteriorly in this horizontal transverse scan.

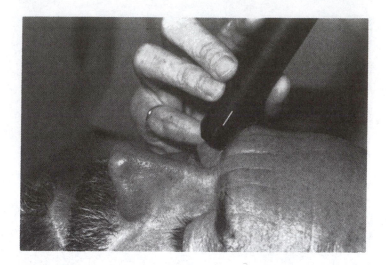

Figure 6.18 Probe moved up toward brow to image inferiorly and anteriorly while patient continues to look down.

Certainly in some situations, the eye must remain closed in order for an ultrasound exam to be performed. Some of these conditions are:

1. Recent trauma, surgery or open wound
2. Infants and children
3. One-eyed patients
4. An examiner who feels uncomfortable with placing the probe directly on the globe

Open Eye Contact Scans

As you can see from the above discussion, the most distinct advantage in performing scans with the eyes open is that you always know exactly what part of the globe is being examined. The additional value in this technique is that with the lids out of the way, more sound energy is being transmitted into the eye. The fat in the lids absorbs and attenuates the sound right from the start, and avoiding this will result in slightly more resolution in the image.

Mini-Immersion Scans

The mini-immersion technique utilizes the same scleral shell device mentioned in the immersion axial eye length section of chapter 4. The reasoning behind this technique is that the optimal area of focus for the B-scan sound beam is between 10 and 30 mm from the probe tip. It is in this focal zone that the area of interest should be imaged.

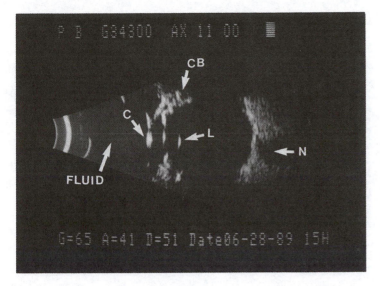

Figure 6.19 "Mini-immersion" scan uses the same scleral axial length. B-probe is gently placed on the top rim of a filled shell. The empty space at the beginning of the scan corresponds to the fluid in the shell. Cornea (C), lens (L), ciliary body (CB), and optic nerve (N) are readily seen. This technique provides greater resolution in the anterior segment.

What if the tissue to be imaged is less than 10 mm from the probe tip—for example, the anterior segment? In the conventional methods of contact scanning, this focal zone of the sound beam would be too far posteriorly, providing a less than optimal image of the anterior segment. In order to bring the tissue into the focal zone, the probe needs to be farther away from the eye. This may be easily accomplished.

The use of a scleral shell filled to the brim with sterile methylcellulose allows the examiner to move the probe tip to the correct position. Now the anterior segment structures will be within the zone of maximum resolution, 10 to 30 mm.

Mini-immersion scans using the scleral shell can be quite useful for imaging anterior segment structures. Moving the probe away from the eye increases the resolution in this part of the eye.

Mini-immersion scans are used in the special case of such pathologies as an iris cyst, ruptured lens capsule, and ciliary body melanoma. On the screen, the image of the eye will be shifted to the right with the anterior segment echoes located approximately in the middle. In the contact method, the anterior segment echo patterns are at the left edge of the screen and the area of interest, the vitreo-retinal interface, is in the center of the screen.

Water Bath Immersion Scans

This technique was the original method by which ophthalmic scans were performed. The patient lies flat while a large drape is glued to the forehead, the side of the nose, the upper cheekbone and the temple areas around the eye. The top of the drape is held in a ring stand. A lid speculum

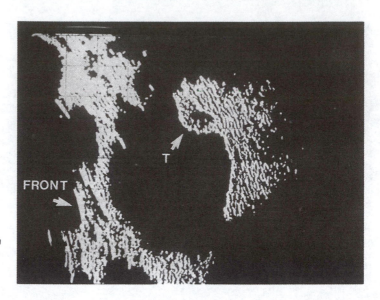

Figure 6.20 This image from a full immersion system has less gray scale, but tumor (T) is clearly imaged.

holds the lids away from the anesthetized cornea and about one liter of saline warmed to body temperature is gently poured into the hopefully watertight setup. With the saline in place, the transducer crystal, which is held by a mechanical apparatus, is lowered into the fluid to the desired depth.

One of the advantages of this system is that it allows the greatest latitude in changing the distance between the transducer and the eye, thereby positioning the tissue within the area of maximum resolution.

Once the transducer is in position in the saline, the examiner must move the crystal back and forth by hand with a small lever. There is no motorized probe here, just the crystal itself. This sweeping motion "paints" an image on a screen which may be photographed if desired. When the scanning has been completed, the drape is punctured to allow the saline to drain into a basin. The speculum is removed and the drape peeled off from around the eye. As complicated and uncomfortable as all this sounds, there are still a few echographers who routinely perform this type of scan. They are accustomed to the setup, and more importantly are used to drawing conclusions from these images.

Although these images have a brightness and crisp clarity about them which is appealing, they do lack gray scale, a term defined in the next section. This makes subtle echoes difficult to differentiate from strong ones.

Describing Echograms

One of the things we talk about when describing B-scans is the relative brightness of the dots or echoes on the screen.

To exhibit a wide variety of intensities from black to white is called gray scale. This range of echo intensities provides additional information about the tissues that reflected the sound.

Bright echoes are called strong reflectors and can also be described as being produced by a strong echo source. Dim echoes therefore come from weak echo sources. Another way of describing these echo patterns is in terms of internal reflectivity. When a lesion is imaged, for example, the appearance of the echoes from inside the tumor are of clinical significance. A tumor with bright echoes is said to have high internal reflectivity. Dim echoes within a tumor indicate low internal reflectivity. Of course, the level of gain will have an effect on whether the echoes are bright or dim,

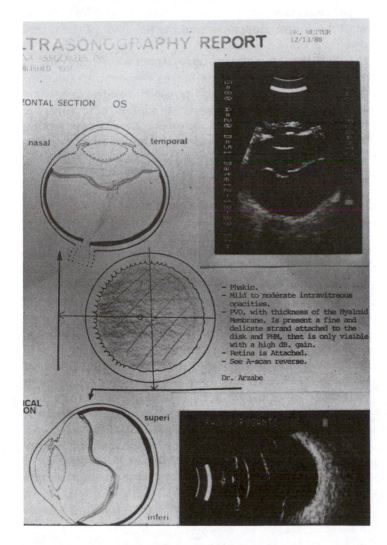

Figure 6.21 One institute's method of reporting ultrasound findings is to combine the echograms with retinal drawings and a written description of the ultrasound exam findings.

so the relative gain value must also be taken into consideration.

An area of a scan may also be referred to as being empty. Two commonly used terms are echolucent or acoustically clear.

There are many additional facets to describing the appearance of B-scan images which vary from one pathology to another. As additional reference materials are studied and pathologies examined, further details will become incorporated into your store of knowledge.

Real Time Scanning

The concept of real time is the idea that when the probe or the eye moves, the image moves at the same time. Another way of stating this is that there is no discernable delay between the probe or eye movement and the behavior of the image on the screen.

Some B-scan instruments have probes whose transducers move relatively slowly. This makes real time evaluations slightly more difficult but still possible once the characteristics of the equipment are understood. For these units, the examiner must slow down the probe movements so that the changes on the screen can be evaluated more readily.

Dynamic Scanning

In addition to the brightness or dimness of echoes, the way they move provides important clues to the nature of the tissue which produced the image. This is the idea behind dynamic scanning. This basically means that while holding the probe stationary, the technician asks the patient to look to a new fixation target then back again. By observing the screen during eye movements, it is possible to evaluate the way in which a structure moves.

For example, when the eye moves, a vitreous membrane whips around on the screen rather quickly. A retinal detachment, however, has an undulating though somewhat restricted motion. In fact, even a total retinal detachment is still attached at the optic nerve and the ora serrata.

Another form of movement that is seen during dynamic scans is the vascularity of a lesion, particularly a melanoma. When the B-scan probe is held still while imaging a large melanoma, it is sometimes possible to see the pulsations of the vascular supply from within the tumor during real time scanning.

A very interesting display of dynamic imaging can be

observed when convection currents move particles around in the vitreous. I have seen blood cells from a fresh hemorrhage in a vitrectomized eye gently moving on their own while the probe is held still. The calcium-lipid opacities that are present in a case of asteroid hyalitis are also known to move on their own as a result of convection currents.

It requires a very sensitive instrument with high gain in order to see a fresh hemorrhage clearly. In a vitrectomized eye this can be even more difficult to see. However, the asteroid bodies are highly reflective due to the presence of calcium; consequently, the image is easily seen even at lowered gain levels.

Labeling Echograms

The only person who knows where the probe was held in relation to the ocular structures during an ultrasound examination is the operator. Therefore, it is their responsibility to properly document and label the images.

Many people have their own abbreviations for labeling scans, and this is fine for the operator's own purposes. When others will see the scan, however, the labeling method becomes more critical. The most thorough method of labeling comes from standardized echography, an examination technique discussed in chapter 7.

The first step in labeling a photo is to note the basic probe orientation as transverse (T) or longitudinal (L). Axial scans are labeled either as vertical axial (VAX) or horizontal axial (HAX). The second step is to label the center of the B-scan image. When the probe is placed horizontally at the 6:00 limbus, and therefore aimed posteriorly at the 12:00 meridian, then the label will be 12:00 P for 12:00 posterior.

It will also be evident from the label that this is a horizontal transverse scan, since that is the only probe position where the 12:00 meridian can be centered in the scan. If the transducer is at the 12:00 meridian in the center of its swing, then it is at the 9:00 point at the top of the screen and the 3:00 area at the bottom of the screen.

Let's say that the probe is now in a vertical orientation, with the center of the probe placed close to the 3:00 equatorial region of the globe as the patient looks away from the probe in extreme gaze. The probe is directed toward the 9:00 meridian, and the sound beam is shifted anteriorly as the probe moves more posteriorly. Since the beam is now directed across the eye at the equator, the label would be 9:00 E for 9:00 equator.

Having an old-fashioned clock with hands can be advantageous to the echographer during the scanning process as well as when thinking about the correct label for an echogram.

PROTOCOL FOR A BASIC EXAM

Being consistent in the examination protocol will speed the learning process. There is so much to think about at the time of the procedure, and it will be quite helpful if the scanning protocol has become a second-nature routine. At least if you scan each patient in the exact same way, you won't have to worry about having forgotten something.

There are six basic probe positions which make up the protocol. If a pathology is detected during the exam, other positions such as the longitudinal and oblique scans should follow.

Position #1 is horizontal transverse with the probe marker directed nasally. The patient is instructed to look up as high as possible and the probe is placed at the 6:00 limbus. As the probe is slowly moved into the lower fornix, the angle of the tip is adjusted so that the probe face stays in contact with the globe. The posterior superior aspect of the globe is imaged with these scans.

Position #2 is vertical transverse with the probe marker directed superiorly. The patient is instructed to look nasally and the probe is placed on the temporal limbus. As the probe is moved into the lateral fornix, the nasal aspect of the globe is examined.

Position #3 is horizontal transverse with the probe marker directed nasally. The patient is directed to look down and the probe is placed on the 12:00 limbus. As the probe is moved into the upper fornix, the inferior aspect of the globe is shown.

Position #4 is vertical transverse with the probe marker directed superiorly. The patient is instructed to look temporally and the probe is placed on the nasal limbus. As the probe is moved into the medial fornix, the temporal aspect of the globe is displayed.

Position #5 is vertical axial with the probe marker directed superiorly. The patient is told to look in primary gaze and the probe is gently placed over the cornea with ample coupling gel. The scan should display the cornea, posterior lens and optic nerve shadow surrounded by orbital fat. The lens echo and the nerve shadow should be centered in the display. Remember that the vertical axial view does not image the macula.

Position #6 is horizontal axial with the probe marker directed nasally. The patient is again fixating in primary gaze and an image of the cornea, lens and posterior structures will be displayed. Center the posterior lens echo and the nerve shadow. This is the scan that will image the macula, just below the nerve shadow on the screen.

If a pathology is noted during this initial exam, then additional scan angles will be necessary in order to determine the extent and exact position of the structures. The pathology or area of interest must be centered in the B-scan display in order to obtain the best resolution of the image. The probe must be positioned in whichever way is required to achieve this goal.

After all the scan angles have been completed, go back and document the ones that best represent the areas of interest. Label the photos in a consistent manner and file them with the patient's chart. If additional ultrasound exams are required at a later date, be certain to pull the photos from the first exam for reference.

ARTIFACTS

As soon as we begin to practice scanning, we notice that there are a wide variety of things happening on the screen which need explanation. A part of interpreting B-scan images is knowing which echoes are real and which echoes are artifacts. An artifact is usually an unwanted echo created by some sort of reverberation or distortion of the sound beam.

Probe Contact

The artifact most familiar to all examiners is one that is produced when the probe is not in full contact with the eye. In this case, the part of the probe which is not coupled

Use copious amounts of gel to avoid probe contact artifacts and to prevent pressing on the globe. Instruct the patient to tell you if you are pushing too hard.

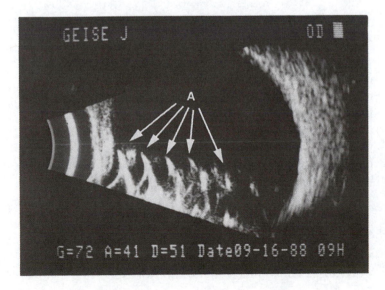

Figure 6.22 The most commonly seen artifact in a B-scan image is that of poor contact of the probe to the ocular surface. Reverberation echoes from the membrane probe tip is what causes these rib-like echoes. Adding more gel will solve the problem.

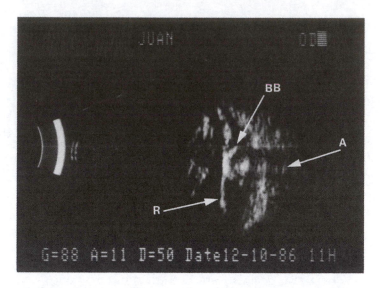

Figure 6.23 *A steel BB from a pellet gun has an unmistakable bright echo from the surface, and a chain of reverberation echoes that follow. In this case, the BB is under the retina (R) and the artifact echoes (A) are seen posterior to the foreign body.*

to the eye with sufficient gel reflects the sound. As a result, part of the scan will have probe tip echoes instead of ocular echoes.

Air Bubbles

Air bubbles are another major source of artifacts. These may be in any of three locations:

1. Inside the probe
2. In the coupling gel
3. In the eye

Air in the Probe

To test for bubbles, hold the B-probe with the tip toward the ceiling. While in the scanning mode, slowly tilt and turn it while observing the screen. Know what air bubbles in the probe look like on the screen so that the probe may be properly maintained.

Ultrasound cannot be transmitted through air bubbles in the probe. Therefore, you must either refill the probe if it is user refillable or contact the manufacturer if it is a factory-filled model. Sometimes if the bubble is small enough, the probe can be positioned in such a way that the bubble will move out of the pathway of the sound and into another part of the probe. This is generally possible if the tail of the probe is held higher than the tip.

Air in the Gel

Micro bubbles in the methylcellulose can be an aggravation. This causes a noisy image in the anterior aspect of the globe, as well as reduced sound energy traveling to the more posterior tissues. When squeezed through the dropper and pressure is released, hundreds of bubbles can be heard being introduced into the solution as air is drawn back into the bottle. In order to prevent this, pop off the dropper tip, throw it away, and replace the cap. In this way, the gel may be poured instead of forced through the tiny tip. Store containers of gel upside down.

Air in the Eye

Air bubbles in the eye may be present due to two reasons:

1. A penetrating injury
2. A pneumatic retinopexy procedure

Penetrating injuries and foreign bodies sometimes introduce air into the eye. Since air does not transmit ultrasound, even small bubbles are strong reflectors of the sound beam and appear on the screen as very bright echoes. In fact, it is often extremely difficult to differentiate an air bubble from a foreign body such as glass or metal. If the bubble in the eye is of sufficient size, a shadow will appear behind it because of the inability of the sound wave to pass through. We must be careful not to mistake these shadows for the optic nerve.

The surgical procedure called pneumatic retinopexy is a process whereby a gas is injected into the eye as a method of reattaching a retina. It is a great challenge to examine a patient who has undergone this procedure. If the air bubble is too large, an ultrasound exam is simply not possible. However, with smaller bubbles, the patient's head may be positioned in such a way that the acoustic section of the B-scan may be directed around the air. Moving the head to a different position will allow another area to be examined. In this way, various areas of the retina may be examined in order to evaluate the relative success of the procedure.

Foreign Bodies

Foreign bodies in the eye present some unique artifactual echoes. In fact, these artifacts are quite useful in making an evaluation of what the material might be. The artifacts created by foreign bodies may be grouped into two categories—those with:

1. Extra echoes generated
2. Lack of echoes posteriorly

Routinely, the gain should be turned down so that the foreign body, which is generally more reflective than ocular structures, may be more easily seen. This is especially valid when looking through the orbital fat. Since the fat itself creates bright echoes, the examiner must scan slowly and carefully with reduced gain in order to detect these objects. Of course with any foreign body patient, or with any trauma for that matter, an X-ray should be taken first in order to look for metallic objects. Speaking of metallic objects, it is not appropriate for a patient with a potentially magnetic foreign body such as steel to be referred for a magnetic resonance imaging (MRI) scan. The high level of magnetism used to create such a scan could easily dislodge the object, or worse yet pull it out of the eye.

Extra Echoes

Extra echoes are generated when foreign material sets up a reverberation of sound energy by its highly reflective nature. A piece of glass or metal can produce extra echoes just behind it due to a principle called reduplication. The key to understanding this is to notice the root word duplicate.

One way to tell which echo is from the real foreign body and which ones are artifacts is to move the probe toward and away from the object. If this is possible, then the examiner will notice on the screen that the actual foreign body echo moves in synchronization with the probe, whereas the reduplication echoes move away from the originating echo at twice the speed.

Before trying this technique on a patient with a recent penetrating injury, you can gain experience by practicing with a convenient, homemade model. Fill a mug halfway with water, preferably bottled water so as to avoid the micro bubbles present in tap water. Place only the very tip of the B-scan probe, or A-scan probe for that matter, into the water and lower the gain enough to visualize a strong reflection from the bottom of the mug.

Carefully observe the echoes and move the probe tip deeper, then lift it slowly while watching the screen. The echo from the bottom of the mug will move in concert with the tip of the probe, but the reduplication echoes will travel across the screen at twice the rate.

I should mention one echo pattern which is unique to only one specific foreign body. Although its characteristic artifact makes the diagnosis easy, in reality it can be a most difficult examination. This is because of the artifact's totally senseless origin. I am referring to the examination of a child who has been shot in the eye with a BB gun.

When the spherical BB enters the eye, it causes considerable damage. Acoustically, a BB presents as a very bright echo followed by a comet tail chain of echoes. This tail is generated by the sound beam reverberating back and forth within the steel sphere.

Pellet guns also take an annual toll on children's eyes. A pellet is made of lead and is softer than steel, changing shape upon impact. Although highly reflective, a pellet generally does not have the same echo pattern as a spherical BB.

Lack of Echoes

An absence of echoes is appropriately called a shadowing artifact. This is caused by the sound beam encountering a total reflector. This means that the sound cannot travel through the material. The optic nerve head is the most common producer of a shadow, but certain foreign bodies can do the same. When the gain is turned down, these shadows become more evident.

CASE STUDIES

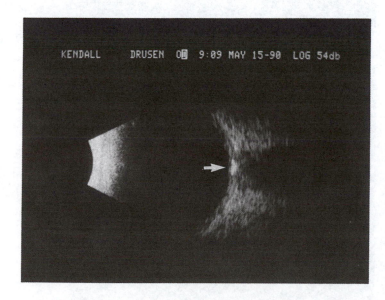

Figure 6.24 The author's own buried disk drusen is a calcium deposit on the optic nerve head. This calcium is so different from ocular tissue that it appears as a foreign body, a bright echo even when the gain is turned way down. The optic nerve shadow is often wider in these cases.

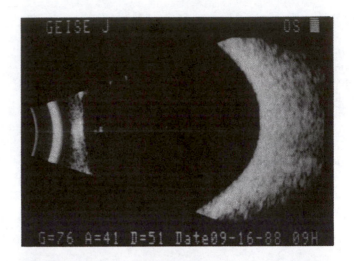

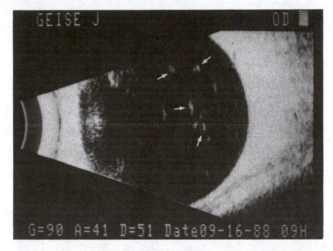

Figure 6.25 A good example of how important it is to vary the gain throughout a B-scan examination. If only the top image were seen (taken at 76 dB), you would think this patient's vitreous was clear. Turning the gain up to the maximum of 90 dB clearly shows the large amount of vitreous opacities and changes in this highly myopic individual.

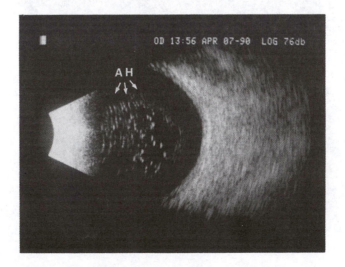

Figure 6.26 A patient with asteroid hyalosis has calcium deposits in the vitreous (AH). The asteroid bodies are clearly visible even with reduced gain, due to their highly reflective nature.

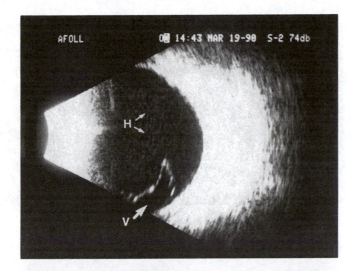

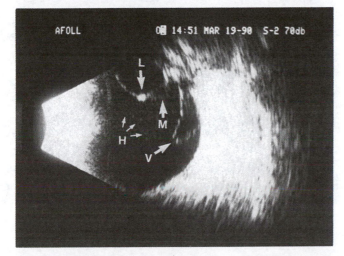

Figure 6.27 Fresh hemorrhage (H) in a vitrectomized eye shows multitude of tiny blood cells suspended in saline. Holding the probe still on the eye allows the examiner to observe convection currents moving the RBCs around in the eye. Residual vitreous (V) is anterior in eye. Lower photo is a longitudinal scan of the same eye with slightly reduced gain and a more anterior view to show posterior lens surface (L), retrolenticular membrane (M), hemorrhage (H) and residual vitreous (V).

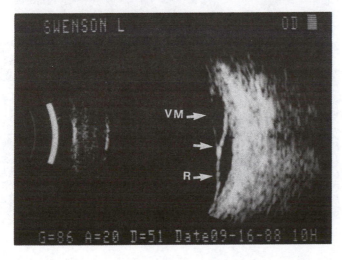

Figure 6.28 Classic case of a traction retinal detachment. Vitreous membrane (VM) has contracted pulling off the retina (R). The point of attachment between the two membranes is shown with the center arrow.

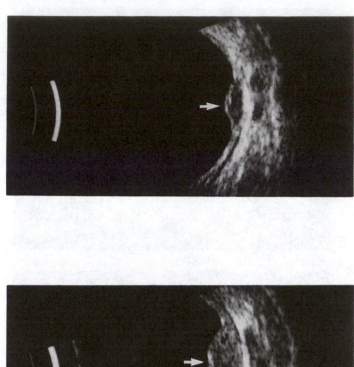

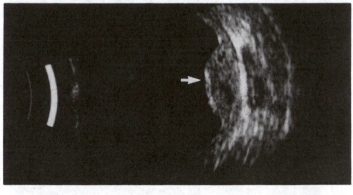

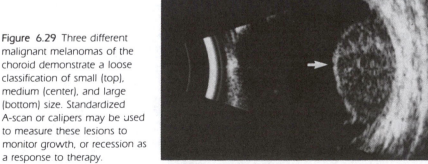

Figure 6.29 Three different malignant melanomas of the choroid demonstrate a loose classification of small (top), medium (center), and large (bottom) size. Standardized A-scan or calipers may be used to measure these lesions to monitor growth, or recession as a response to therapy.

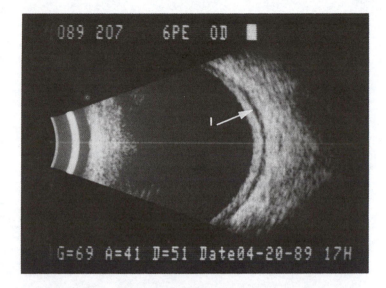

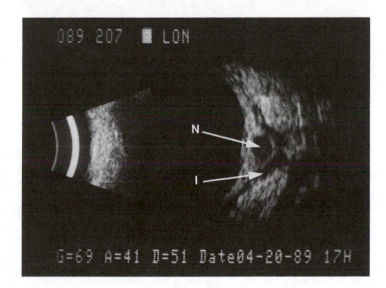

Figure 6.30 The patient has posterior scleritis, an inflammation of the episcleral space (I). Lower photo shows a transverse section of the optic nerve (N) demonstrating the inflammation's (I) involvement of the nerve.

CONCLUDING REMARKS

The role of the ultrasound exam is to provide one piece of the diagnostic puzzle. Clinical observations combined with other tests and imaging methods such as X-ray, CT, and MRI will complete the array of information available. B-scans are such an important tool since they are very revealing, relatively easy to perform, significantly less expensive than other imaging methods, and do not expose the patient to radiation or magnetism.

Be a team player. Read up on the various conditions for which you are performing an ultrasound exam. Understand the disease process so that the echographic findings will make more sense to you.

CHAPTER 7

Standardized Echography

WHAT IS STANDARDIZED ECHOGRAPHY?

The term standardized echography has a very specific meaning. It describes a specialized method of performing echographic examinations of the eye and orbit. The exam is a combination of B-scan and a unique type of A-scan referred to as standardized. This A-scan is not merely for making measurements, although it is often used in this way. The primary use of standardized A-scan is to perform tissue characterizations and thereby aid the examiner in making a diagnosis of a specific condition.

The three components of the standardized echography method are:

1. Standardized A-scan
2. Contact B-scan
3. Standardized examination techniques

The use of doppler to study ocular blood flow is also included as a diagnostic mode, though it is used infrequently.

Please recall the concepts set forth in chapter 1 regarding the production of echoes by the interfaces between dissimilar tissues. These ideas may be dramatically expanded upon when utilizing standardized diagnostic A-scan. With this technique, the actual cellular characteristics of structures may be acoustically evaluated.

One example of the use of standardized echography is to differentiate choroidal hemangioma from choroidal melanoma. On B-scan, these tumors may have similar contours, both being dome-shaped lesions of the choroid. Differences between the two can sometimes be shown in B-mode— melanomas have somewhat dimmer internal echoes while hemangiomas are brighter. This difference is more evident with standardized A-scan, where a hemangioma will have taller internal echoes than a melanoma.

The interpretation of relative brightness of echoes on the B-scan is dependent upon the subjective evaluation of the

Since only specific instruments can be labeled as standardized, be very careful about the terminology. There is a difference between what some call "close to standardized" and truly standardized.

Standardized diagnostic A-scan, contact B-scan, standardized examination techniques, and the occasional use of doppler are components of the standardized echography method.

examiner, not to mention the coincidental setting of the gain. A higher gain can make a melanoma's internal echoes look as bright as a hemangioma. How then can we differentiate these tumors?

With standardized A-scan, there is a characteristic difference between the internal echo pattern from these two. A histology slide of each will in fact show a marked difference in the cellular structure. The hemangioma contains stagnant blood within vasular spaces, whereas the melanoma cells are small and uniformly distributed. The assortment of cell sizes and types in the hemangioma provides many interfaces of dissimilar tissues, and hence many reasonably tall echoes. The melanoma, on the other hand, with its uniform composition provides few large interfaces to produce strong echoes. Therefore, the melanoma is said to have low internal reflectivity. Evaluation of these echo patterns is referred to as quantitative echography.

How is it that standardized A-scan can show this difference better than the B-scan? The key point is that when performing a standardized A-scan, the gain value is set at precisely the same value for every patient (called Tissue Sensitivity). In addition, it is difficult to judge whether one B-scan echo is brighter than another, while it is easy to see if one A-scan echo is taller than another.

The following sections will discuss the specific characteristics of the equipment used which classify that equipment as standardized.

UNIQUE EQUIPMENT CHARACTERISTICS

There are three components of a standardized A-scan setup:

1. An amplifier with specific characteristics
2. An A-scan probe of unique frequency and beam shape
3. A tissue model for determining Tissue Sensitivity

Amplifier Design

The amplifier in any ultrasound instrument—whether for ocular applications or otherwise—is designed in such a way that the specific tissues to be imaged will appear clearly. This is the reason why an abdominal scanner does not work well for the eyes and vice versa. In the standardized amplifier, there are precise values which determine how the echoes will appear on the screen. Additionally, these values are exactly the same from one standardized instrument to the other.

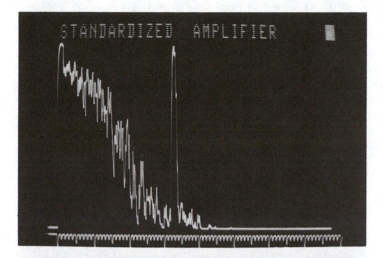

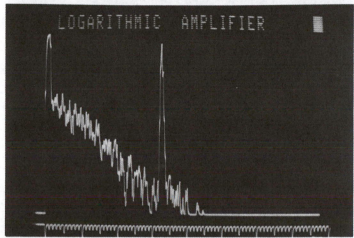

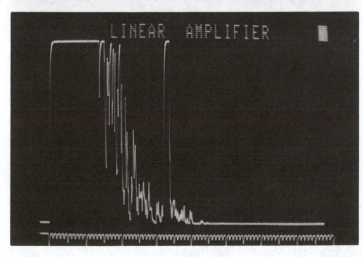

Figure 7.1 These pictures show the same frozen A-scan from a tissue model (TM) with different types of amplification applied. They demonstrate why specific amplifier characteristics are imperative for diagnostic consistency. The logarithmic amplifier compresses the echoes so that there is not so much difference from one to the other. In contrast, the linear amplifier exaggerates the differences making low echoes lower and high echoes higher.

When you look at axial length A-scans produced by various instruments, you will see that each instrument displays the A-scan in a slightly different manner. Some show tall, thin echoes while others show shorter, wider ones. For measuring axial lengths, this is adequate and acceptable. However, in making a diagnosis it would be better if every instrument produced comparable images.

The amplifiers in standardized instruments are so exactly the same that a patient can be examined, for example, in Los Angeles and then soon afterwards in Buenos Aires and both examiners will obtain the same A-scan image on their standardized equipment.

Probe Design

The A-scan probe used in this method also has two precise characteristics, frequency and beam shape.

Frequency

Standardized A-scan probes are a bit lower in frequency than most axial length and B-scan probes. The standardized probe operates at 8 MHz and the sound beam is parallel, not focused like the others

The frequency of a standardized A-scan probe is always 8 megahertz (8 MHz). This is eight million cycles of sound per second. This frequency is slightly lower than the 10 MHz used in the B-scan and most axial length biometry probes.

Beam Shape

The sound beam which emanates from this 8 MHz probe is not focused as in the B-scan and biometry probes. Instead, it is a parallel beam. This parallel beam is very useful in determining perpendicularity. It also allows all the tissues which come into the beam's path to be subjected to the same amount of sound. This probe does not have an internal fixation light and has a characteristic stainless steel barrel.

Tissue Models

In the early days of standardized echography, perhaps twenty years ago or more, the original sample tissue model was a solution of citrated blood. Now of course there is a man-made tissue sample produced in Europe which meets special requirements. It is used to determine the appropriate level of gain when utilizing standardized A-scan for diagnosis. This tissue model (TM) is a small metal canister containing a transparent, rubbery substance in which tiny glass beads are suspended.

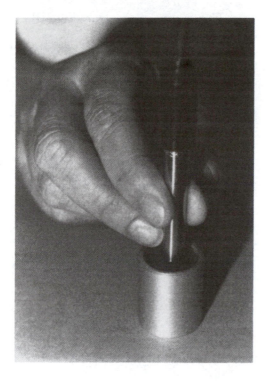

Figure 7.2 This is the tissue model used in standardized echography. An echogram is obtained from the TM and the gain is adjusted to produce a specific pattern. This gain value will then be the one used for most examinations.

For every probe/instrument combination, the TM is used to determine the tissue sensitivity (T). This sensitivity is a value of gain required to make the A-scan image of the TM appear on the screen in a specific way. The probe is placed on the top of the model with a few drops of saline or water for coupling. The degree of display magnification must be "orbit," a setting on the equipment, which compresses the image horizontally. This helps make the TM echo pattern easier to interpret.

When using the model, begin with the gain or sensitivity turned up high. There will be a series of tall echoes from within the TM. Slowly turn down the gain while maintaining perpendicularity with the bottom of the container. This will be evident by the sharply rising tall echo produced by this strong reflector. As the gain is lowered, the echoes from inside the TM will decrease in amplitude. The goal is to adjust the gain until the chain of internal echoes appears as a diagonal. The diagonal appearance separates the echogram into two echo-free triangles of the same size.

A gain value that is too high will produce a larger echo-free triangle under the diagonal than above it. Too little gain will produce a lower triangle smaller than the upper one. Each person in the world who performs standardized echography verifies the tissue sensitivity value in the same

Only the tissue model made in Europe is accepted as the standard for this technique. It is manufactured with very specific characteristics to allow for determination of the proper gain value used in each examination.

way. This is one of the benefits of the standardization of echographic techniques.

If the console or probe is repaired or changed, the tissue sensitivity value must again be determined. In fact, it is recommended that this value be verified frequently, at least once each month to check for changes in the probe. As the probe ages, the transducer becomes less sensitive and the tissue sensitivity value will increase slightly.

Once the correct image pattern is obtained and the gain value displayed, as in the newer freeze frame units, take a photograph of the scan of the tissue model and keep it handy for reference.

For all basic examinations, the same value of tissue sensitivity will be used for each and every patient. When a more precise measurement of a structure is required, then a lower sensitivity will be used in order to display more clearly the echoes to be measured. In some situations, a higher value should be employed such as $T + 6$ dB, which is the tissue sensitivity plus six decibels. The higher figure is used when examining the vitreous for subtle pathologies such as a fresh hemorrhage or inflammatory cells in the case of endophthalmitis. Sometimes a value of $T + 8$ dB or even as high as $T + 10$ dB may be used for this purpose.

STANDARDIZED INSTRUMENTS

There are three instrument models which are currently standardized as per Karl C. Ossoinig, MD, of the University of Iowa, who began developing this technique twenty-five years ago. One of the three instruments, the Kretztechnik 7200 MA, which was manufactured in Austria, is no longer made. However, there are many of these still in use around the world. These units are a hundred percent analog in that the image cannot be frozen on the screen. Other points about the Kretz, as it is usually called, are that it requires daily, if not hourly manual calibration and there are no on-screen electronic measuring cursors. Measurement of the echogram is made by hand holding a caliper device against the Polaroid image. A distance in microseconds is then converted to millimeters by consulting a chart of various velocities.

The other two instruments which currently are standardized are the Ophthascan 'S' and the Ophthascan Mini-A, both made by Alcon/Biophysic. These units have the ability to freeze the image and to apply electronic measuring gates. Of these two units, the 'S' unit is a B-scan also and both its A-scan and B-scan images have a slight delay of movement on the screen. This makes it somewhat more difficult for the examiner to evaluate the dynamic or kinetic characteristics of structures. The ability to visualize the spontaneous echospike movements that are characteristic of the vascularity of a melanoma, for example, is compromised. The Mini-A, however, has a faster image display rate and the vascularity is readily seen.

NONSTANDARDIZED INSTRUMENTS

Instruments which do not have officially standardized A-scan amplifiers are called diagnostic A-scan. The "generic" diagnostic A-scans from various manufacturers may have some similarities to the truly standardized systems but cannot be used to compare clinical images. If a true standardized A-scan is desired, be careful to verify the fact that the unit has been approved by an authority who can attest to its standardization.

PREPARING THE PATIENT

The preparation of the patient for standardized echography is similar to all other types of scans. Position them comfortably with their head near the instrument's screen and provide fellow eye fixation.

STANDARDIZED EXAMINATION TECHNIQUES

The standardized techniques of scanning are very similar to the ones outlined in the chapter on B-scans. Again, the examination is to be performed in the same way each time.

Probe Positions

The first probe position is the 6:00 limbus with the probe angled posteriorly. Shifting the probe into the fornix, the sound beam sweeps along one meridian from posterior to anterior.

The second probe position is toward the temporal side of the eye. On the right eye, this is the 7:30 position. On the left eye, the first position toward the temple is 4:30. The probe is again shifted from the limbus into the fornix, thereby scanning the superotemporal meridian.

The standardized examination method is similar to that described in the B-scan chapter. Be methodical and consistent; it's hard to forget something if you perform a task in the same way every time.

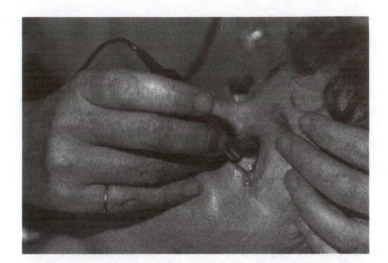

Figure 7.3 Just as in B-scan, the initial probe position is the 6:00 limbus with the patient looking away, imaging the posterior portion of the 12:00 meridian, labeled 12:00 P.

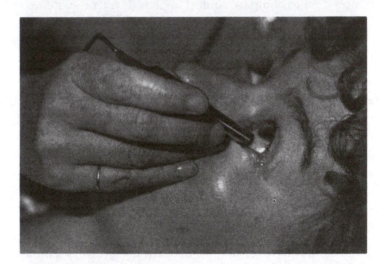

Figure 7.4 The probe is now halfway to the fornix, imaging the 12:00 meridian at about the equator of the globe, labeled 12:00 E.

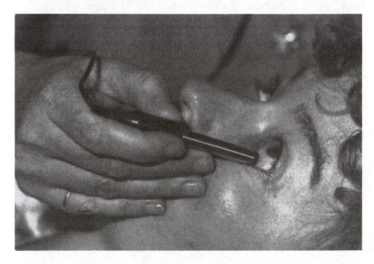

Figure 7.5 The probe is now in the fornix, imaging very anteriorly along the 12:00 meridian, labeled 12:00 CB for ciliary body.

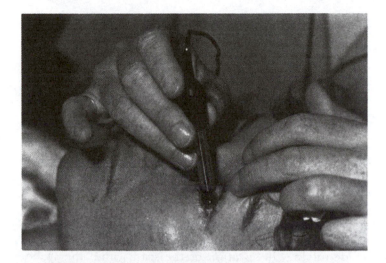

Figure 7.6 The 3:00 meridian is being examined posteriorly, 3:00 P.

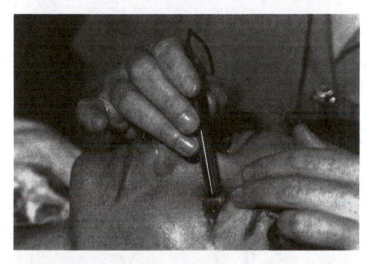

Figure 7.7 As the probe moves toward the inner canthus, the area being examined becomes 3:00 EP, between the equator and posterior pole.

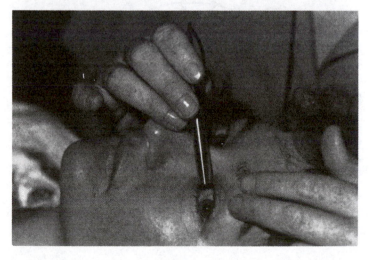

Figure 7.8 The most extreme position of the probe now images 3:00 CB for ciliary body region.

The third position is at 9:00 on the right eye and at 3:00 on the left.

The probe positions continue in this fashion until all eight meridians have been examined. As with B-scans, the patient is primarily instructed to look away from the probe.

Labeling of Echograms

The method for labeling standardized A-scan photos is similar to the way in which diagnostic B-scans are labeled. The area that is being imaged—opposite the probe—determines how the photo is labeled. In addition to the clock hour notation, an identification of the anterior/posterior aspect of the meridian may also be made.

Standardized echography provides a thorough method for identifying the location of the scan within the globe. From anterior to posterior, these positions are labeled:

AX   Axial (probe on cornea)
CB   Ciliary body
O   Ora serrata
EA   Equator toward anterior
E   Equator
EP   Equator toward posterior
PE   Posterior toward equator
P   Posterior pole

The eight primary clock hour positions for both eyes are:

6:00   7:30   9:00   10:30   12:00   1:30   3:00   4:30

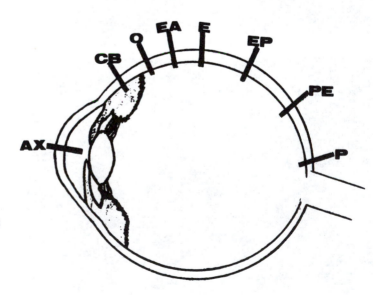

Figure 7.9 Keep a copy of this labeling diagram available during every examination for assistance in determining the area being imaged.

(Drawing courtesy of Sandra Frazier Byrne.)

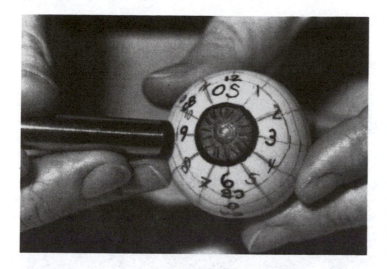

Figure 7.10 This clever labeling tool is a prototype made by Stewart Martin, CRA to enable him to grasp the concepts more quickly. There is a left and a right eye model, so that the probe may be actually placed on the model helping the examiner to visualize the area of the eye being imaged.

As an example, imagine that the probe is placed on the right eye in the 9:00 position, directed toward the 3:00 meridian. The probe is also positioned halfway between the limbus and the fornix, about at the equator. A photo of this A-scan would be labeled 3:00 E.

The probe is moved to the next position on the right eye, the 10:30 orientation. In its first position on the limbus, the probe is directed toward the posterior pole at 4:30. This photo would be labeled 4:30 P. For additional examples, see the section titled Labeling Echograms in chapter 6.

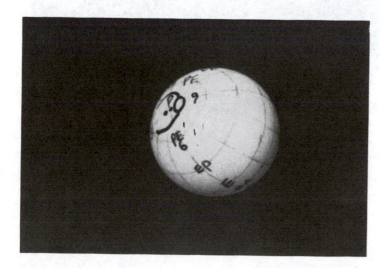

Figure 7.11 The back of Stewart Martin's eye model showing the posterior labels, macula, and optic disk. For additional information, contact Mr. Martin c/o Carol Grocki, 415 East 78th St., #1D, New York, NY 10021.

CASE STUDIES

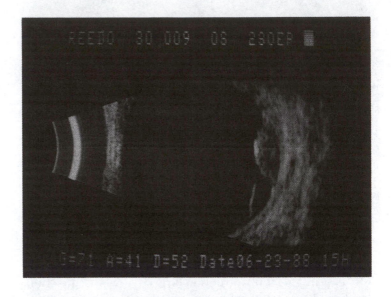

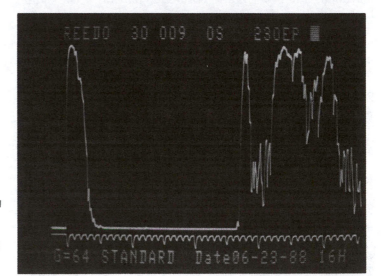

Figure 7.12 Top photo shows a classic B-scan of a choroidal melanoma with adjacent retinal detachment. Bottom photo is standardized A-scan of same lesion with characteristic strong echo from tumor surface and weaker signals from inside.

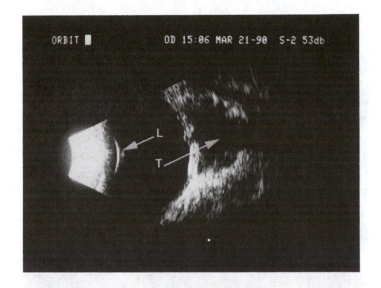

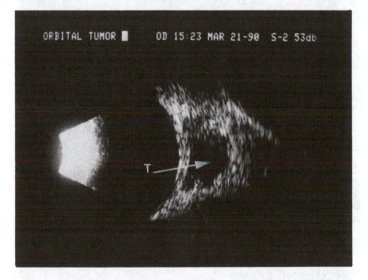

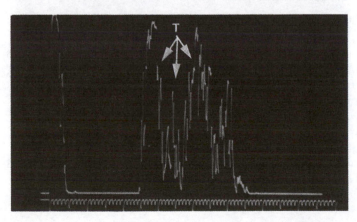

Figure 7.13 Top photo shows axial view of an orbital tumor (T) that involves the optic nerve. The lens is visible (L). Center photo shows a different probe angle of the same lesion. Bottom photo is standardized A-scan from tumor showing irregular structure and medium reflectivity. This tumor is a metastatic carcinoma.

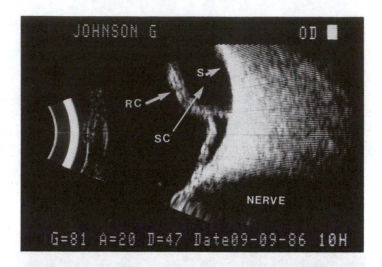

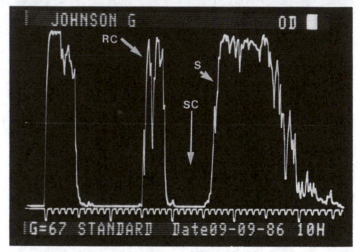

Figure 7.14 This retinal and choroidal (RC) detachment shows how retinas insert to the disk and choroids do not. In the upper edge of the scan, the RC layer is off, showing sclera (S) behind the subchoroidal space (SC). Since this is a longitudinal scan, the optic nerve is at the bottom of the echogram. Note on the A-scan that the sub-choroidal space is echo-free, indicating a detachment rather than a tumor, and a serous rather than a hemorrhagic detachment.

CONCLUDING REMARKS

Standardized echography is a sophisticated diagnostic technique which can be learned by applying the basic principles and by using very specific examination procedures. It is highly recommended that a student receive formal training in this technique and that they observe the work of echographers proficient in this method.

Standardized echography is the ultrasound technique which is being used for the Collaborative Ocular Melanoma Study (COMS) currently under way in North America. Forty-two ophthalmic centers throughout the United States and Canada are participating in this trial and have at least one echographer certified in the method. This work is being directed by Ms. Sandra Frazier Byrne, Adjunct Assistant Professor of Ophthalmology and Director of Echography at the University of Miami, Bascom Palmer Eye Institute, Miami, Florida. By using the standardized echography technique, echographers at these varied centers have learned to communicate in a universal echographic language to provide accurate results in order to better serve the patient's needs. The ultimate goal of this study is to determine the optimal course of management for patients with ocular choroidal melanoma.

CHAPTER 8

Ocular Relationships and IOL Calculations

OCULAR RELATIONSHIPS

The purpose of this chapter is to acquaint the reader with the effects that corneal power, lens power, and overall length of the eye have on the eye's refraction. It is important to understand these ocular relationships so that the array of numbers used during the entire process of calculating an IOL power makes sense, is of significant value, and correlates with the patient's history and spectacle refraction.

When an IOL power is given in this chapter, unless otherwise noted it refers to the power required to produce a postoperative result of emmetropia or plano when implanting an intraocular lens.

Effect of Axial Length

First, let's examine how changes in the axial length of the eye will affect the refraction. In Figure 8.1, all three corneal powers and natural lens powers are the same; only the lengths differ. The center drawing shows an average eye length of 23 mm, with the resultant refraction of plano. The top example shows that in an eye one millimeter shorter at 22 mm, the refraction is now hyperopic at +3 D. On the bottom, the myopic example is demonstrated by increasing the length by one millimeter to 24 mm producing a refraction of −3 D.

One millimeter in axial length equals three diopters of refraction.

The accepted rule is that 1 mm = 3 D. This is a worst case situation. Often the effect is slightly less than 3 D.

Effect of Corneal Power

Next, the effect of changes in the corneal refraction will be shown. In Figure 8.2, all three eyes have the same axial length and natural lens power; only the keratometry readings are different. The center drawing is again the plano

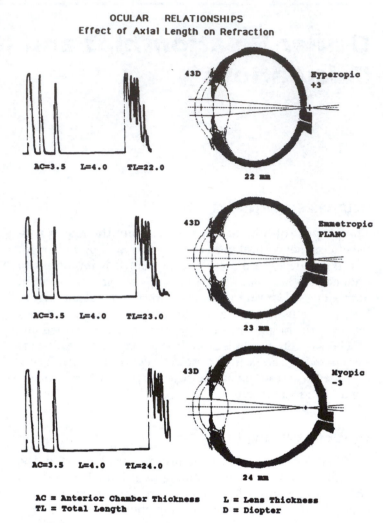

OCULAR RELATIONSHIPS
Effect of Axial Length on Refraction

AC=3.5   L=4.0   TL=22.0

43D   Hyperopic +3   22 mm

AC=3.5   L=4.0   TL=23.0

43D   Emmetropic PLANO   23 mm

AC=3.5   L=4.0   TL=24.0

43D   Myopic -3   24 mm

AC = Anterior Chamber Thickness   L = Lens Thickness
TL = Total Length   D = Diopter

Figure 8.1 Relationship between axial length and refraction when corneal power remains the same.

Always measure postoperative keratometry first when troubleshooting a less than desirable result. Remember that the cornea provides two-thirds of the refractive power of the eye. Next measure the post-op axial length.

example with a length of 23 mm and an average K reading of 44 D. The top drawing is a hyperopic eye because the cornea is now much flatter at 41 D. The bottom eye illustrates the myopic effect when the keratometry value becomes steeper at 47 D. Since the cornea represents approximately two-thirds of the refractive power of the eye, it is very important to understand the significance of this measurement when evaluating pre- and postoperative refractions.

Effect of Natural Lens Power

Finally, there is one last aspect to consider. The overall refraction of the eye is of course affected by the power of the natural lens itself. In Figure 8.3, all three eyes have

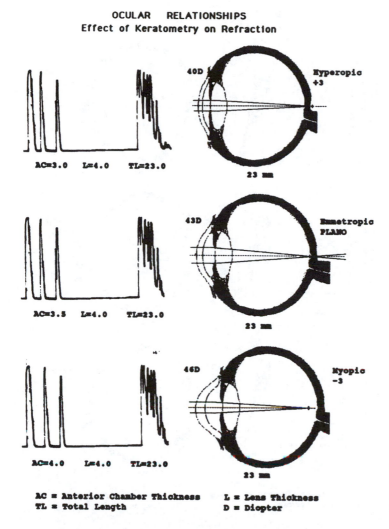

OCULAR RELATIONSHIPS
Effect of Keratometry on Refraction

40D   Hyperopic +3
AC=3.0   L=4.0   TL=23.0
23 mm

43D   Emmetropic PLANO
AC=3.5   L=4.0   TL=23.0
23 mm

46D   Myopic -3
AC=4.0   L=4.0   TL=23.0
23 mm

AC = Anterior Chamber Thickness   L = Lens Thickness
TL = Total Length   D = Diopter

Figure 8.2 Relationship between corneal power and refraction when axial length remains the same.

the same axial length and corneal powers. The only difference between them is the power of the natural lens, indicated in the drawing by varying thicknesses. The center eye shows the plano example, while the top one shows the effect of a natural lens with less than average power, resulting in the hyperopic refraction. The bottom drawing illustrates a very common occurrence in patients who are developing cataracts. Often the lens becomes swollen, with the changes brought on by the cataract. This causes the lens to increase in power, thereby producing a myopic effect, even though the patient may never have been myopic before. This condition is referred to as cataract induced myopia. Patients sometimes say that they have acquired a feeling of "second sight." Their vision has actually improved since

As a cataract develops, it often swells. This increased lens thickness has more refractive power and patients often experience a renewed ability to see things close up. This is called cataract induced myopia.

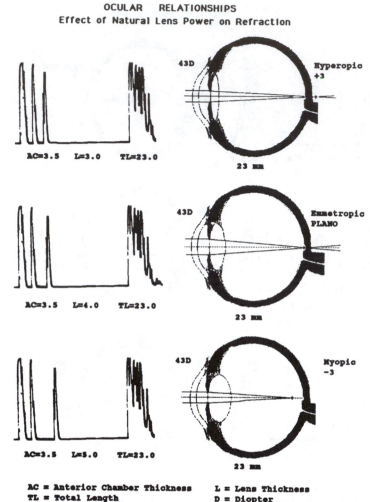

OCULAR   RELATIONSHIPS
Effect of Natural Lens Power on Refraction

Figure 8.3 Relationship of lens power (thickness) and refraction when corneal power and axial length remain the same.

they developed the cataract, because they can now read without their glasses, even though the image may be foggy.

Effect of IOL Position

Another postoperative troubleshooting measurement is the IOL depth. Compare the measured post-op value to the IOL company's predicted value. A post-op value smaller than predicted will result in extra myopia for the patient. Deeper than planned IOLs produce extra hyperopia

When the postoperative result is more myopic than anticipated, this could indicate that the IOL's final location was more anterior than expected. Conversely, if the final refraction is more hyperopic, it may be that the position was slightly more posterior than planned. When the same surgeon intends to operate on a patient's fellow eye and implant the same type of lens which he used in the first eye, it can be of benefit to know where the first IOL ended up.

Making Sense of the Numbers

When performing calculations on an eye having average values for both K readings and axial length, one should expect an average emmetropic posterior chamber IOL power in the range of 18 D to 20 D.

When an unusually low IOL power such as 10 D is calculated, it should be correlated with the patient's preoperative refraction. In this case, one would expect a myopic eye. Conversely, an unusually high IOL power such as 25 D should correlate with a hyperopic patient. The same is true for the ultrasonic axial length. Just because the A-scan reading may be an unusually large number, for example 28 mm, this doesn't necessarily mean that it is wrong. Look at the oldest known refraction for the patient and it should be myopic. Conversely, if a very short axial length is determined, verify it by looking for a hyperopic pre-cataract refraction. You should expect to calculate a correspondingly higher than normal power for the IOL.

Mother Nature of course thrives on exceptions and the following are examples demonstrating the thought process whereby "making sense of it all" is shown.

When preparing to calculate an IOL power write the numbers down and make sure they make sense. Does the axial length fit with the keratometry? What about the refraction, does it correlate with the length?

Example #1

A patient is measured for IOL calculations and the axial length is 25 mm. At first, one might expect a myopic eye, since we know that the average eye length is approximately 23 mm. When the patient is questioned about eyeglasses, they respond that they have never worn any and that they had excellent vision prior to developing the cataract. How can this be? What other part of the eye's refractive system could have as unusual a value in the opposite direction? When looking at the K readings, it is seen that the patient has quite flat Ks which counteract the unusually long eye. This verifies the fact that for this patient, an axial length measurement of 25 mm makes sense.

Let's follow this thought further. Just by evaluating the axial length alone, we could make an initial guess as to what the patient's refraction might be. Since it is 2 mm longer than the average length of 23 mm, and knowing that 1 mm = 3 D, we would assume that the patient's refraction would be in the neighborhood of -6 D (2×3 D = 6 D). Realizing that a longer than normal eye is myopic, the refraction is labeled with a minus sign. Since the K readings for this patient are so much flatter than average, approximately 39 or 40 D, this has canceled out the effect of the long eye and the patient's refraction of plano now makes sense.

Example #2

At the other extreme, what about a patient who has a pre-cataract refraction of −6 D? What would be expected when measuring the length? The patient has average K readings, so we anticipate an axial length of approximately 25 mm. This estimate is made by taking the average length of 23 mm and adding 1 mm for each 3 D of myopia. Knowing this, and expecting a longer than average length, how can the patient measure only 24 mm? Working backward from this length, our guess is that the refraction is −3 D. But the actual refraction of the patient is really −6 D.

The measured axial length doesn't make sense. Or does it? What else about the eye's optical system could account for that extra 3 D of myopia? What about the natural lens power? It appears that this patient has some myopic effects from the changes in the structure of the lens caused by the development of the cataract. Now, after examining all of the pieces of the puzzle, the refraction of −6 D does make sense.

A second ending to this story could be that the patient's K readings are steeper than average (47 D) which would increase the myopic effect.

It should therefore be expected that the combination of numbers (K readings, axial length, and IOL power) makes sense for each and every eye examined and, possibly, provides an idea of the effect of cataract development on the eye's refractive error.

Summary of Relationships

In summary, remember the average values for the ocular relationships and use them to correlate the measured results to the patient's medical history:

Average axial length =   23 mm*
Average keratometry reading =   44 D
Effect of 1 mm in diopters =   3 D
Average emmetropic IOL power = 19 D for posterior
                                                        chamber lenses

---

*The U.S. average eye length is 23.5, but for the sake of making the arithmetic simpler I chose to use the value 23 mm here.

Average emmetropic IOL power = 17 D for anterior
chamber lenses

IOL CALCULATIONS

There are both simple and complex methods for determining the power of IOLs that are appropriate for each
patient. One of the earliest formulas was the clinical history
method. This formula states that D = 18 + (1.25 × Rx).
D is the IOL power in diopters which would be required
to produce emmetropia, and Rx is the patient's preoperative spectacle refraction. The reason why more sophisticated methods were developed was that this method was
only as good as the accuracy of the patient's oldest known
refraction.

As was brought out earlier in this chapter, the changes
that occur within the lens can alter a patient's refraction.
When the patient's history is not known, it is difficult to
know what percentage of their present refraction was induced
by the cataract. Therefore, an incentive existed to create a
more scientific formula.

Major errors have been made
by simply entering incorrect
data into a formula. Make
certain the entered values are
correct.

Early Theoretical Formulas

The first of the formulas to be developed were very long
and complicated and were based on the theories of optics.
The equations contained values for the index of refraction
for the cornea, aqueous, and so on. It was mandatory that
a small hand-held, programmable calculator be used to perform these mathematical contortions. The theoretical formulas were named for the physicians who developed the
various subtle variations.

Some of the physicians who developed the first formulas
were Binkhorst, Collenbrander, Shammas, and Fydorov.
The Collenbrander formula was modified by Hoffer and is
called Collenbrander/Hoffer.

Input Data

The three primary pieces of input data for these theoretical
formulas are:

1. Axial length
2. Average keratometry reading
3. Anticipated postoperative anterior chamber depth

Regression

The regression formula was developed by doctors Sanders, Retzlaff and Kraff, hence the name SRK formula. When this formula was first created, it offered a unique answer to the challenge of predicting the correct IOL power: it worked backward from the theoretical formulas. The regression-type formulas may also be called empirical formulas.

In basic terms, theoretical formulas theorized that the IOL power determination should be based on preoperative measurements and estimations of the postoperative anterior chamber depth of the implant. The SRK formula, in a sense, asked a computer to come up with a formula based on the actual postoperative results. In other words, it asked the computer this question: "What would the formula have to have been in order for the postoperative results to have turned out the way they did?" Working backward from known results is the basis for the name regression formula.

This formula has an added benefit in that it is so simple a pocket calculator can handle the job instead of having to buy the more expensive one that theoretical formulas require. The drawback of the SRK formula, however, is that it is less accurate than the theoretical formulas in the case of abnormally long eyes.

The SRK group came up with a modification which decreased the calculated IOL power for myopic eyes and increased the power for hyperopic ones. This version of the formula is called SRK II, and it was popular for a number of years. The latest supplement is called SRK-T; the T stands for theoretical, since this formula now incorporates some of the features of the original theoretical methods. (This information has been published in 1990 by SLACK Incorporated. The title is *Lens Implant Power Calculation* and its authors are John Retzlaff, MD, Donald R. Sanders, MD, PhD and Manus Kraff, MD.)

Input Data

The three pieces of input data which are required by the regression formulas are:

1. Axial length
2. Average keratometry reading
3. A-constant

The A-constant is a pure number which has no unit like diopters or millimeters. It is a value which essentially expresses the relative position of the IOL in the eye. This value is initially determined by the IOL manufacturer and may be later modified by surgeons to conform to their personal surgical techniques. The first A-constant values for various styles of IOL were obtained through the work of clinical trial physicians. These physicians provided data to the IOL company statisticians regarding their patients' preoperative and postoperative conditions.

A Little of Both

The Holladay formula is a more recent development. Even though it has been around for a few years, it has been slow in gaining popularity due to the relative ease of use of the more familiar SRK formulas. Over time, however, physicians encountered situations in which the original SRK formula and even the SRK II were awkward. These included patients' postoperative results still being slightly more myopic and hyperopic than anticipated and small changes in axial length causing large changes in predicted IOL power. The Holladay formula, which is a combination of aspects of the theoretical as well as regression schools of thought, is gathering more enthusiasm as its reputation increases.

One of the really nice features of the Holladay formula is that there are flags in its computerized program which alert the operator when data are out of the normal range. This helps prevent postoperative surprises which are due to inaccurate preoperative measurements. When calculations are made using this program, a message on the screen will ask the operator to ascertain if the out-of-range entered value is actually correct. This will hopefully prompt the person to think about the ocular relationships and correlate the values with the patient's history.

Input Data

With the Holladay formula, the first two input data are the same as in the SRKs. Only the third is different:

1. Axial length
2. Average K reading
3. Surgeon factor

Comparative Calculations

With eyes that have normal preoperative measurements, which of course represent the majority of cases, all of the formulas will yield very similar results. It is in the long myopic eyes and the short hyperopic ones where the formulas begin to diverge. It is impossible, however, to say

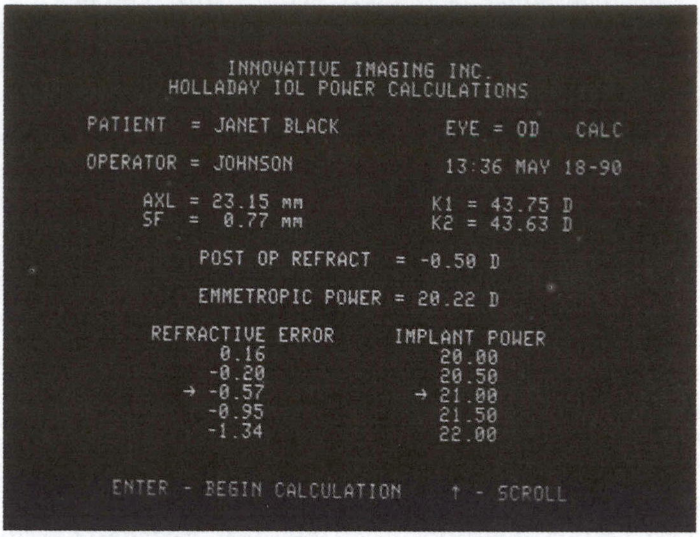

Figure 8.4 Sample IOL calculation using the Holladay formula.

that someone should use one or another of the formulas. Choosing a formula is a personal preference on the part of the physician. Many physicians are still using the original SRK formula and have had so much experience over the years that they have adopted personal correction factors. In effect, they have modified the formula to meet their surgical needs. And this is more than appropriate. What is important is having a formula which produces good surgical results.

CONCLUDING REMARKS

Every once in awhile there is a surprise postoperative result which confuses everyone. This can precipitate a decision by the surgeon to switch to a completely different formula. It is recommended that formulas not be abandoned too hastily. Many cases should be reviewed before such a step is taken. The puzzle may in fact be solved by performing postoperative measurements.

If, however, someone is beginning a new practice and is deciding on their first IOL formula, or if a physician insists on trying a new formula, I would recommened Holladay or SRK-T. A nice feature of the Holladay is that it seems to have combined the best features of theoretical and regression ideas with a relatively easy format. Many articles have been written over the years comparing formulas, and these may be found in various cataract surgery journals. My goal here is simply to provide an idea of how the formulas work and what input data are required.

CHAPTER 9

THE NEXT STEP

WHERE TO GO FROM HERE

There are many roads to walk down that will further your knowledge of ophthalmic echography. Reading is only one part of the learning process. Each examination of a patient, each discussion of a case with technicians or physicians, each new question you have and the research required to find the answer expands the foundation of your knowledge making you a better echographer. In this chapter, I will provide a few guideposts that you may find useful.

Keep up-to-date with what is happening. Join a society, attend lectures and courses. Meet others in your area who are performing similar tasks. Learn from your colleagues

Practice

Virtually every echographic examination, whether of normal eyes or of those possessing pathological conditions, offers new opportunities for learning. Even after years of practice, there are new observations to be made when carefully evaluating echo patterns from actual cases. If you can find a time when the patient load is low, ask the physician if you may examine cases that may have conditions from which you could learn. Of course this would be at no charge to, and with the permission of, the patient. This will help you to keep active in the three-dimensional thought process.

Courses

Formal courses are not in abundance, so watch carefully for announcements in journals and in the mail. Often, brochures describing technician courses are mailed to a doctor's office marked "For the technician of." These sometimes get lost in the shuffle. Ask the person who sorts the mail to pass these brochures on to you.

JCAHPO-sponsored courses are offered in conjunction with the American Academy of Ophthalmology in the fall of each year. Be sure to contact JCAHPO in Saint Paul, MN, for information, (612) 770–9775.

Occasionally, physicians or institutes sponsor courses during the year. One that has been held each spring for the last fifteen years or so is under the direction of Yale Fisher, MD, at the Manhattan Eye, Ear and Throat Hospital in New York City. This Saturday course, titled "Contact B- and A-scan Ultrasonography for the Clinician," is directed primarily toward diagnostic B-scan and is usually sold out prior to the actual course date. Watch for announcements in journals, or contact the continuing medical education department at the hospital for further information, (212) 838–9200.

Courses specifically covering the techniques and understanding of standardized echography, under the direction of Karl C. Ossoinig, MD, are held throughout the year at different locations in the United States and abroad. These courses are usually three days in duration, sometimes five. To contact people and societies who can provide course dates and locations, refer to a later section in this chapter concerning organizations.

It would be beneficial to have an understanding of basic ultrasound techniques prior to attending any standardized echography course as these are generally more advanced in nature. Please realize that if standardized echography is to be studied, you should not expect to become an expert after just one session. It would be advisable to attend several, perhaps once each year.

Courses from which you might obtain new knowledge that will help you in performing echographic examinations do not have to be exclusively about echography. Local eye institutes, and physician and technician societies also sponsor seminars. I have given lectures and workshops at a number of well-organized meetings that included A-scan with IOL calculation at a cataract surgery symposium and diagnostic B-scan at a retinal meeting. These ultrasound lectures and workshops in conjunction with others directed toward an ophthalmic specialty are very beneficial and provide a forum for discussing interrelated subjects. An increased awareness of a specific disease process greatly benefits the echographer's understanding of echograms.

Observation

Observing others is a vital part of learning. It is certainly the way I learn best. The skill level reached through attending courses, lectures, and workshops has a limit which can only be extended through practice. When this is combined with the observation of fellow echographers, the expansion

It is so important to observe a master echographer. If you want to excel, convince your employer that you should receive some hands-on clinical training under the supervision of an experienced technician or physician. You'll be amazed by what you will learn.

of your abilities is continuous. When I observe others performing echography, I always gain something new, even if it is an idea of how not to do something.

Organizations

There are three organizations devoted specifically to ophthalmic ultrasound. Two are American and one is international. These are:

1. American Society of Ophthalmic Ultrasound (ASOU)
2. American Association of Ophthalmic Standardized Echography (AAOSE)
3. Societas Internationalis pro Diagnostica Ultrasonica in Ophthalmologia (SIDUO)—the International Society for Diagnostic Ultrasound in Ophthalmology

ASOU

The ASOU is a group that furthers knowledge and use of diagnostic B-scan and other related imaging methods such as CT and MRI used in ophthalmology. Several members of this society are involved in very interesting ultrasound research. The person to contact is the executive secretary/treasurer:

> Ms. Lois Hart, RDMS
> Massachusetts Eye and Ear Infirmary
> Department of Ophthalmic Ultrasound
> 243 Charles Street
> Boston, MA 02114

Dues are $25 per year and a newsletter announces meetings and items of interest. The society has an annual evening meeting at the AAO where scientific papers are presented and reports are made.

AAOSE

The AAOSE is a society whose emphasis is on standardized echography—the special form of combining B-scan with a specifically designed A-scan to characterize tissues. Dues include membership in SIDUO. The person to contact is:

> Karl C. Ossoinig, MD
> University of Iowa Hospitals
> Department of Ophthalmic Echography
> Iowa City, IA 52242

Each year at the AAO, the society has a formal scientific meeting in which papers are presented and questions are answered. Their newsletter announces upcoming courses.

SIDUO

The international group, SIDUO, meets every two years in a different part of the world. Four days are filled from morning to night with the presentation of scientific papers from every possible point of view and with exciting new ideas. Even if attending one of the congresses may not be feasible right now (although occasionally they are held in the United States) it would still be of benefit to become a member of the society. Their publications are educational, and you would be able to order the printed proceedings of each scientific meeting. The dues are $15 (US) per year and a money order should be sent to the treasurer of the society:

> H. John Shammas, MD
> 3510 Century Blvd.
> Lynwood, CA 90262

Certification

In case you wondered about the letters after Ms. Hart's name, mentioned earlier, RDMS stands for Registered Diagnostic Medical Sonographer. This certification is part of the much larger group that works with those who perform abdominal, cardiovascular, and other types of diagnostic ultrasound. There is an extensive study program associated with certification and each specialty has a separate qualifying examination. The governing group is:

> Association for Registered Diagnostic
>   Medical Sonographers (ARDMS)
> 32 East Hollister Street
> Cincinnati, OH 45219
> (513) 721–6662

If you would like to know more about the ophthalmology certification, contact the association. Currently, there are about 45 people certified for ophthalmology, whereas there are over 16,000 people registered in other specialties.

Reading

The most recent and most thorough information specifically relating to echography was published in 1989. This appears as the long chapter "Diagnostic Ophthalmic Ultra-sound" in the first of a three-volume set titled *Retina*. The authors of the chapter are Ronald L. Green, MD, and Sandra Frazier Byrne. The editor in chief is Stephen J. Ryan, MD, and the publisher is C. V. Mosby of St. Louis, MO. This chapter provides an in-depth discussion of techniques and diagnoses for many ocular disorders. It is highly recommended reading.

In 1984, the *Atlas of Ophthalmic Ultrasonography and Biometry* by H. John Shammas, MD, was published by Mosby. This 321-page, large-sized volume provides an easy-to-read format with text on the left and photos on the right. Basic principles are reviewed, as well as an overview of many of the ocular pathologies we encounter in echography.

A very interesting text that compares echographic findings with photographs of the actual pathology sections was published in 1987 by Springer-Verlag in New York. The title is *Macroscopic Ocular Pathology—An Atlas Including Correlations With Standardized Echography*. The authors are F.H. Stefani and G. Hasenfratz from West Germany. I found it to be a fascinating presentation, especially for those of us who rarely have the opportunity to examine a patient with an indirect ophthalmoscope, let alone are able to see the actual post-enucleation pathology sections.

Future Developments

The challenge of the future is to increase our ability to create, document, store, and transmit ultrasound images. Computer disk storage and processing is beginning to become available. Years ago we used to imagine having a network of computers linked with a group of echography gurus so that they could assist others throughout the world. We dreamed about being able to simultaneously observe both the probe on the eye and the actual echogram at a remote location, thereby assisting with the diagnosis and management of patients.

With the escalation of computer technology, this idea seems less farfetched each year. One computer use that is becoming a reality is a data base of patient scans and diagnoses. Jackson Coleman, MD, of Cornell University, has been working with the study of patterns of frequency shift in echoes reflected from tumors and other structures. Dr. Coleman has also been working with three-dimensional imaging of the eye. Very exciting things are indeed on the horizon for the field of ophthalmic echography.

CONCLUDING REMARKS

I would like to thank you, the reader, for taking the time to read and to expand your knowledge of the field of echography. I will be delighted to receive comments, questions, ideas, and suggestions, and to incorporate the many shared ideas in my teaching and writing.

My best advice is to never stop asking questions; never quit striving to expand your knowledge and improve your technique.

Index

Page numbers in *italics* refer to illustrations